PET/CT in
Clinical Practice

PET/CT in Clinical Practice

T.B. Lynch

With Contributions by:

James Clarke
Gary Cook
Simon Hughes
Mark Love
Chris Marshall
Stephen Vallely
Lorraine Wilson
Sandra Woods

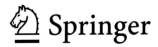 Springer

T.B. Lynch, MB, BSc, MSc, MRCP, FRCR
Senior Lecturer
Department of Medicine
Queen's University
Belfast
and
Lead Nuclear Medicine Physician and Consultant Radiologist
Nuclear Medicine and Radiology Department
The Northern Ireland Cancer Centre
Belfast
UK

British Library Cataloguing in Publication Data
Lynch, T. B.
  PET/CT in clinical practice
  1. Cancer—Tomography   2. Computerized axial tomography
  3. Tomography, Emission
  I. Title
  616.9'940757
ISBN-13: 9781846284304
ISBN-10: 1846284309

Library of Congress Control Number: 2006927787

ISBN-10: 1-84628-430-9   eISBN-10: 1-84628-504-6
ISBN-13: 978-1-84628-430-4 eISBN-13: 978-1-84628-504-2

Printed on acid-free paper.

9 8 7 6 5 4 3 2 1

Springer Science+Business Media
springer.com

Preface

The combination of functional metabolic information and anatomical data has been available since 2001, when the combined PET/CT scanner was introduced. This technology has had a significant impact on many medical disciplines, including cardiology and neurology, but undoubtedly the greatest impact has been in the field of oncological imaging. It is the ability of PET/CT to accurately identify the anatomical location of abnormal metabolic activity that has revolutionized the detection and staging of many tumors.

With this in mind, this small book has been written. The focus is on the role of PET/CT in cancers of the lung, esophagus, colon, and head and neck. The text also considers the impact of PET/CT on lymphoma, melanoma, and cancers of the reproductive system.

Each chapter outlines the relevant staging system and illustrates how PET/CT can best be deployed in tumor evaluation. A large number of PET and PET/CT images are included in each cancer type, with illustrative case studies used to aid teaching points. The presentation is basic, with many representative images of each cancer type, as well as a comprehensive review of normal PET/CT findings and commonly seen variants (Chapter 9). Chapter 1 provides a general introduction to cellular biology and Chapter 10 provides a brief overview of the physics involved in PET/CT.

This book does not consider the whole range of positron emitters available but focuses only on the role of F-18 fluorodeoxyglucose (FDG). The emphasis throughout has been to create an easy-to-read, accessible text, suitable for anyone interested in an introduction to PET/CT. The author hopes this book will provide a useful introduction to this fascinating, rapidly evolving and hugely influential area of medical imaging.

I would like to sincerely thank the Springer staff for its significant input in the preparation of this book, in particular

Melissa Morton and Eva Senior. I would also like to recognize the exhaustive efforts made by Barbara Chernow, and the contributions made by my colleagues in providing text and images, for which they deserve much credit. Finally I would like to dedicate this book to the memory of Gloria, Hugh, and Rosemary.

T.B. Lynch
Northern Ireland Cancer Centre
Belfast City Hospital
October 2006

Contents

Contributors

James Clarke, FFRCRI, FRCS
Department of Nuclear Medicine, Royal Victoria Hospital, Belfast, UK (Chapter 5)

Gary Cook MD, FRCR, FRCP
Department of Nuclear Medicine, Royal Marsden Hospital, London, UK (Chapter 4)

Simon Hughes, FRCR
Department of Nuclear Medicine, Royal Victoria Hospital, Belfast, UK (Chapter 6)

Mark Love, FRCR, FRCS
Department of Radiology, Royal Victoria Hospital, Belfast, UK (Chapter 4)

Chris Marshall, MD
Head of Radioisotopes, Nothern Ireland Medical Physics Agency, Belfast, UK (Chapter 10)

Stephen Vallely, MD, FRCR, MRCP
Department of Nuclear Medicine, Belfast City Hospital, Belfast, UK (Chapter 7)

Lorraine Wilson, BSc, MSc, MRCP
Department of Nuclear Medicine, The Blackrock Clinic, Dublin, Ireland (Chapter 8)

Sandra Woods
Senior Clinical Scientist, Northern Ireland Medical Physics Agency, Belfast, UK (Chapter 10)

Chapter 1
Introduction

This introduction outlines what this book is about and just as importantly what it is NOT about. The fact is, if you want to stay up to date in medicine, you cannot avoid PET/CT. This discipline is exploding at the moment with new scanners being placed in hospitals all over the United States and throughout Europe. You can run but you can't hide from the impact this new technology is making, particularly within oncology but increasingly in many other medical disciplines.

This handbook offers a starting point for anyone interested in learning a little about PET/CT. The text is relatively straightforward and the book is stacked full of interesting images. We assume no background knowledge of the subject and give an enthusiastic, well informed basic introduction. This is PET/CT 1.1, nothing more and nothing less.

If you already have an interest in this field and a working knowledge of PET/CT, I would recommend buying a copy of Jadvar and Parker's excellent book *Clinical PET and PET/CT* (ISBN: 1-85233-838-5). Their small handbook is a great stepping stone for those who have attained a basic grasp of the subject, and the authors delve more deeply into the science of PET than I can in this book. No department should be without Sally Barrington's excellent, award-winning new PET/CT atlas. There are many other fine textbooks worthy of mention but few are aimed at individuals with little or no background in nuclear medicine and PET/CT.

Are you a radiologist or nuclear medicine physician with little or no experience with PET/CT? Are you experiencing more and more exposure to this subject at multidisciplinary meetings?

Are you a physician or surgeon with an interest in any of the following cancers? *Lung, Lymphoma, Gastro-oesophageal, Colorectal, Head and neck, Melanoma or Genitourinary.*

Are you about to acquire a PET/CT scanner in your hospital?

Are you a resident or medical student keen to learn about the latest technology?

If the answer to any of these is yes, then this book can provide a useful starting point for you.

The aim is to inform readers about the role of PET/CT in the big six cancers: lung, lymphoma, esophageal, colorectal, head/neck, and melanoma. Brief mention is also made of gynecological, and testicular cancer. The physics involved is skipped over lightly (Chapter 10), and an outline of normal and common variant uptake is included in Chapter 9.

Each big six chapter contains a summary of the associated staging scheme. The most common staging system used is the TNM (tumor, node, metastases); this will be familiar to most readers. In some tumor types, other staging schemes are used and these will be outlined within the relevant chapter. I hope to show how PET/CT fits into the staging process, where it is best used and, just as importantly, where it should not be used. This book contains a significant number of images and case scenarios to illustrate the use of PET/CT.

Throughout this book reference is made to PET/CT, but this is a misnomer. What I really mean is FDG-PET. FDG is only one of many radioactive tracers that can be used in PET/CT, but it the one most widely used in oncology imaging and the only tracer that is discussed in this book. For all intents and purposes, throughout this book, PET/CT means FDG-PET/CT.

WHAT IS PET AND PET/CT?

PET (Positron Emission Tomography) is an imaging modality that identifies the presence of a metabolically active tumor within the body after injecting a radioactive substance called FDG. This localizes within areas of metabolic activity around the body and emits radiation that allows us to image the distribution of metabolism, a so-called functional image. A CT (computed tomography) scan uses X-rays to provide an anatomical image of the patient. A PET/CT machine is a single device that combines both modalities to produce an image that shows the metabolic functional information from the PET image and the anatomical information from the CT scan. The resultant data is displayed as a combined, or fused, PET/CT image.

Top Tip

PET + CT = PET/CT
Metabolic function + Anatomy = Fused image

Before we begin to discuss the nature of PET/CT imaging, I would like to consider the basic cellular metabolism involved in tumor growth. From a simplistic point of view, tumors want to divide, multiply, grow, and invade their surroundings. If possible they will spread to distant sites and repeat the same process.

To achieve this objective, the tumor must have an energy source capable of fueling this division and growth. Otto Warburg, a German Biochemist noted more than 80 years ago that many tumors use glucose as their primary energy substrate for this process. As tumors grow, they often become starved of oxygen and, therefore, anerobic metabolism of glucose becomes easier to sustain than aerobic metabolism within the Tricarboxylic acid cycle. The result of this is increased utilization of glucose within tumor cells in relation to most other cells.

Of course normal cells also use glucose for their day-to-day function but in general the glucose uptake in most normal cells is relatively low. Active tumors tend to have a much greater metabolic rate than most normal cells and consequently use considerably more glucose.

Some cells within the body can use several different energy sources to fulfil their metabolic needs. Cardiac muscle, for example, preferentially uses free fatty acids as an energy source, but it can also use glucose, lipids, or amino acids if required. As a result, the glucose uptake within the heart varies among people and can change considerably within an individual over a short period in relation to the blood glucose. Brain cells do not have the ability to use any fuel other than glucose and consequently the glucose activity within the brain is always high.

> **Top Tip**
> Tumor cells often use more glucose than normal cells.

In a fasting state, most body tissues (with the exception of the brain) actually use free fatty acids as their preferred energy source. After a glucose rich meal, these will temporarily switch from free fatty acids to glucose metabolism because they are under the influence of rising insulin levels.

The uptake of glucose into cells is facilitated by transmembrane proteins called glucose transporters. At least 12 different glucose transporters have been identified and are known as GLUT 1, GLUT 2, and so on. When the glucose molecule enters the cell, it is phosphorylated under the influence of the enzyme hexokinase. The resultant compound is called glucose-6-phosphate. Under normal circumstances, the glucose-6-phosphate will undergo further enzymatic change and be converted into energy, a process called glycolysis. Alternatively the glucose-6-phosphate may be stored as a future energy reserve in the form of glycogen, a pathway called glycogensis, or it may possibly be converted into either lipid or protein form.

The increased energy demands of a dividing tumor cell necessitate a faster and more efficient delivery of glucose to allow rapid growth. As the cellular division and growth proceed, the tumor cell finds ingenious ways of meeting its energy requirements. Firstly, the cell will increase the number of transmembrane GLUT transporters to aid glucose delivery. If this is still insufficient to meet demand, the cell can increase the rate of phosphorylation by upgrading hexokinase activity. The resultant effect is that many tumor cells demonstrate marked increases in glucose metabolism when compared to normal cells (see Figure 1.1).

Metabolic Changes in Tumor Cells
Increased cell division
Increased glucose turnover
Increased activity of glucose transporters
Increased hexokinase activity

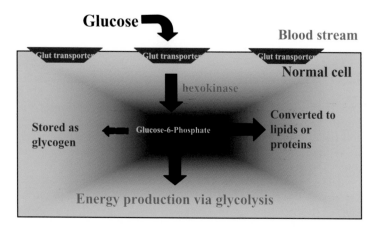

FIGURE 1.1. Uptake and metabolism of glucose in a normal cell

HOW CAN WE IMAGE GLUCOSE METABOLISM?

Fluro-deoxy-glucose (FDG) is an analog of glucose that is labeled to the radioactive positron emitter Flourine-18. The FDG is injected intravenously and is taken up by normal and tumor cells alike in a fashion similar to glucose. In fact, FDG and glucose actively compete with each other for cellular uptake and transport using the GLUT transporters.

When within a cell FDG will be converted into FDG-6-phosphate under the action of hexokinase. The pattern of uptake and phosphorylation being identical for both glucose and FDG. Beyond this point however their pathways diverge, whereas glucose is converted into either energy or stored as glycogen, FDG undergoes no further reaction and by in large remains trapped in the cell.

FDG is a radioactive substance and emits radioactive particles called positrons (see Chapter 10 for a basic description of the physics involved in PET/CT and a brief mention of some other positron emitters and their possible medical usage). FDG has a half-life of approximately two hours, meaning that the amount of radioactivity within the body will halve every two hours. Practically speaking. this means that approximately 3% of injected activity will remain in the patient after 10 hours (or 5 half-lives).

The distribution of radioactivity within the body can be imaged using a specialized camera called a PET scanner. The resultant image gives a picture of the areas of the body which have FDG (and therefore glucose) uptake. The intense accumulation of FDG within many tumor cells allows those cells to be identified when compared to the less intense uptake in normal cells. Patients are imaged in the fasting state because most normal cells will continue to use free fatty acids as their energy substrate. FDG will primarily be taken up into tumor cells as these cells often lack the ability to effectively use other substrates for energy production (see Figure 1.2). Figure 1.2 is a PET scan showing the normal distribution of glucose (as identified by FDG uptake). This image is called the maximum intensity projection image or MIP and is the 2 dimensional representation of the accumulation of FDG uptake in the body as a whole. The appearances are sometimes likened to that of a glass man.

We can see that the brain has intense uptake, with less marked uptake in the heart, liver, and spleen. What we also see is intense uptake in the renal system, kidneys, ureters, and bladder. As you will be aware, normal individuals do not excrete glucose through the renal system, but FDG is excreted renally. We must remember that FDG is not glucose; it is only an analogue of glucose, and it

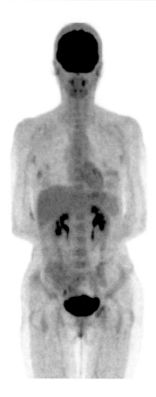

FIGURE 1.2. The distribution of FDG within a normal individual (MIP).

is handled in a different way than normal glucose. Whereas most normal glucose is freely filtered within the renal glomeruli and rapidly reabsorbed by the nephron, the FDG filtered is poorly reabsorbed and a large proportion is excreted in the urine.

Top Tip
FDG distribution reflects the glucose metabolism in the body (except for the renal system).

As explained earlier the cardiac uptake of glucose can be variable. Figure 1.3 shows a different patient with more intense cardiac uptake (which can indicate a recent glucose meal). In addition this patient shows bilateral uptake in the neck muscles, a common finding in tense patients and representative of physiological glucose uptake due to muscular contraction.

FIGURE 1.3. Normal MIP with more intense cardiac and physiological neck muscle uptake.

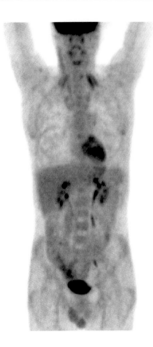

Figures 1.4–1.8 are examples of abnormal scans, with the abnormality highlighted by arrows.

It is difficult to believe that the patient in Figure 1.8 had a normal CT scan of the chest, abdomen, and pelvis. The patient had a previous history of colorectal cancer and had a recent rise in tumor markers. The PET/CT scan revealed multiple bony deposits as well as an unsuspected subcapsular liver secondary.

Figure 1.9 is an axial image through one of the bony vertebral metastases identified on the MIP image seen in Figure 1.8. The CT component is viewed in the top left hand corner and the PET in the top right. The more intense the FDG (or glucose) uptake the blacker it appears on the PET scan. The fused PET/CT scan is seen in the bottom left hand corner of the image. This image combines both the anatomical data from the CT and the metabolic data from the PET; the color scale chosen shows the FDG uptake as increasingly orange with increasing activity. Technology allows the PET and CT images to be viewed separately or as a combined PET/CT or "fused" image. In this case the normal appearance of the CT scan hides the fact that a metastatic deposit exits in the vertebral body. This patient had multiple osseous metastases that were not identified by CT and only some of which were found on a subsequent MRI scan.

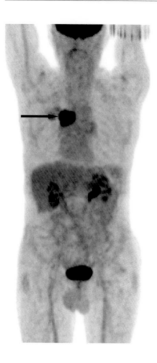

FIGURE 1.4. A FDG positive right hilar squamous cell carcinoma.

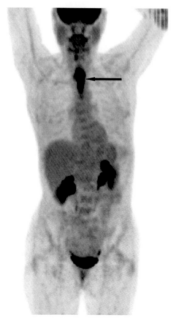

FIGURE 1.5. An upper oesophageal squamous cell cancer.

FIGURE 1.6. A nasopharyngeal lymphoma with bilateral neck node involvement.

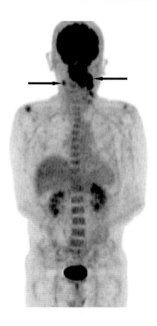

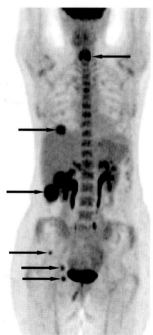

FIGURE 1.7. Recurrent colorectal cancer with metabolically active deposits in the liver and right hemipelvis. The uptake in the neck is due to a coincidental thyroiditis.

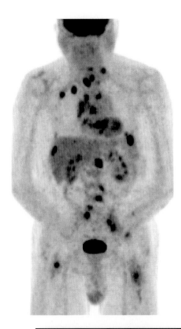

FIGURE 1.8. Multiple bony metastatic deposits.

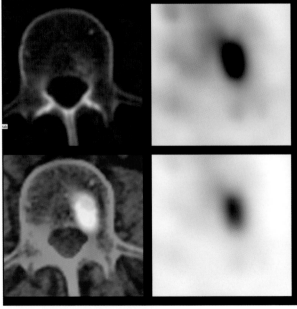

FIGURE 1.9. An axial image through one of the bony vertebral metastases seen in Figure 1.7.

NORMAL SCANNING PROTOCOL AND DESCRIPTION OF IMAGING SEQUENCE

Patients should arrive at the nuclear medicine department having fasted for at least four hours. This ensures that most tissues are using free fatty acids as their energy source. Diabetic patients are advised to take their normal insulin or medication prior to arriving at the department.

After the staff have made all the necessary patient checks, including correct patient identification and a check of blood glucose level, the injection of radioactive FDG can take place. The patient is advised to lie still for approximately 45 minutes to allow the FDG time to accumulate in metabolically active cells. Any unnecessary patient movement during this uptake period can result in muscular uptake which can cause confusion with later scan interpretation. Patients who are tense during this time often show physiological uptake within the muscles of the neck. Some other patterns of normal uptake are illustrated below and a list of normal and variant uptake is found at the end of this chapter.

Following the uptake period, the patient is taken into the scanning room and lies supine on the table. A picture of a GE discovery lightspeed PET/CT scanner is shown in Figure 1.10. The CT scan is performed first, normally without intravenous contrast but increasingly after the administration of oral contrast to outline the normal bowel. The CT scan is normally carried out from the base of skull to mid-thigh level, the so-called half body scan. The reasons for this are:

- Brain metastases are difficult to detect using FDG as any brain lesion must have an intensity greater than or less than the surrounding brain tissue to be identified.
- Generally speaking, few tumors that have metastatic deposits that disseminate to the distal lower limbs.
- There is a decreased radiation burden to the patient.
- There is a considerable amount of time saved if we do not have to perform a whole body scan.

Whole body scans are carried out in some patient groups. For example, patients with melanoma have a whole body scan from skull vertex to feet. This is because of the widespread and unpredictable lymphatic dissemination that characterises this disease. A similar problem is encountered with the pattern of disease spread in non-Hodgkin's lymphoma, which often requires a larger scanning volume.

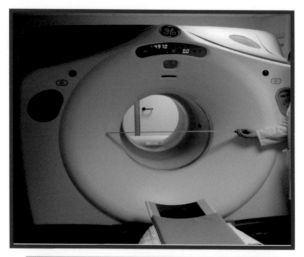

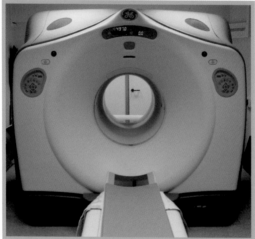

FIGURE 1.10. GE PET/CT scanner.

Patients with head and neck disease often have scans that include the entire skull, and patients with soft tissue sarcomas may also require additional views. After the CT images are acquired (which only takes a minute or so when using a modern multislice scanner), the patient is then scanned again using the PET component of the machine. The detectors on the PET scanner can identify radioactive emissions from the FDG within the body. A ring of detectors surrounds the patient. This ring is approximately 15 cm long, and images are therefore acquired in blocks of 15 cm from the base of the skull to mid-thigh. In most individuals, this area is covered in about 5 blocks (approximately 75 cm); taller or shorter individuals will take more or less imaging time. The time required for each 15 cm image of the patient is between 3 and 5 minutes. This means that the PET component of the study can take at least 45 minutes to acquire. Any patient movement during this time will degrade the quality of the images obtained.

After the PET scan has been acquired the patient is free to go but is given warnings about exposure to individuals during the next few hours as the radioactivity decays and is excreted from the body.

Figure 1.11 is another axial image in a patient with lymphoma who had received chemotherapy. The clinician wanted to out rule residual active disease. As you can see, there is a metabolically active soft tissue mass in the left axilla which was later shown to be residual follicular non-Hodgkin's lymphoma.

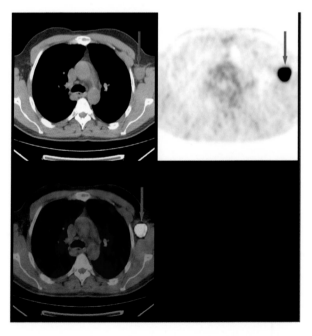

FIGURE 1.11. An axial image. Top left: CT image showing a 3 cm nodal mass in the left axilla (red arrow); top right: PET scan showing intense uptake; bottom left: fused PET/CT image shows active nodal recurrence in a patient with previous follicular non-Hodgkin's lymphoma.

Standardized Uptake Value

A semiquantitative method is available to calculate the intensity of FDG uptake within a range of interest on the PET scan. This value is called the Standardized Uptake Value (SUV) and takes account of such factors as injected activity, patient weight, and time from injection. Simply speaking, the SUV assumes that if there is an even distribution of radioactivity throughout the body the SUV would be measured as 1. Obviously this is not the case, but we can calculate the relative uptake within different parts of the body and relate them to each other. An area with an SUV of 5 means this area has five times the average uptake. Certain modifications can be made to the SUV calculation to take into account, for example, the patient's body fat (since FDG is not generally taken up into fatty tissue).

The SUV allows comparisons to be made between different parts of the body and between different scans on the same patient over a period of time. It must be emphasized that the SUV is only a semiquantitative measurement and can vary considerably with changes in patient's plasma glucose levels.

Many clinicians prefer to avoid numbers and simply use visual interpretation to compare the intensity of one area to another suing the background blood pool as a guide to normality. There is evidence to suggest that both methods are equally accurate. Figures 1.12 and 1.13 demonstrate the change in intensity of an esophageal tumor following chemotherapy

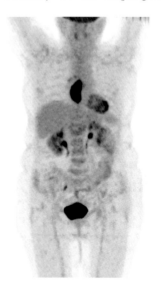

FIGURE 1.12. Pretherapy SUV 15.

FIGURE 1.13. Posttheray SUV 2.

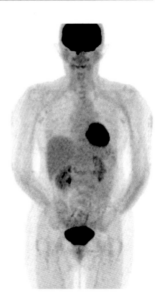

the maximum SUV had decreased from 15 pretherapy to 2 post-therapy. Recent literature would suggest a response of this magnitude correlates with a better prognostic outcome.

List of Normal and Variant Uptake
See Chapter 9 for a list and illustrations of common patterns of normal uptake and examples of some variant uptake.

NOTE ON ILLUSTRATIONS
Please note that throughout this book the above orientation is used on all axial images. Top left corner is the CT image; bottom left the fused PET/CT and top right is the PET image. There are however some images that contain a fourth image in the bottom right corner. This appears very similar to the PET image above it. The bottom right image when present is the nonattenuated correction image and is slightly different from the PET image above it (top right) which represents an attenuation corrected PET image, (see Chapter 10 for a more detailed explanation).

Chapter 2
Lung Cancer

The incidence of lung cancer has been on the rise since the early 1930s, and lung cancer is now by far the most common cancer in the Western world. It has been the leading cause of cancer death in males for more than half a century. In recent years, the number of female smokers has relatively increased and now more than 30% of all new cases are women. In addition, the rate of cigarette consumption has been on a sharp rise in Eastern and developing countries.

The mortality of lung cancer has barely improved over the past 40 years, with an overall 5-year survival rate of less than 10%.

Pathological subtype	Frequency
Squamous cell cancer	35–45%
Adenocarcinoma	15–50% (large regional variation)
Large cell carcinoma	10%
Mixed forms	10–20%
Others: carcinoid, sarcoma etc.	2%
Small cell carcinoma	20% (considered disseminated at presentation in most cases)

Lung cancer is staged using the TNM system which has been shown to a correlate with prognosis. The classification is given in Table 2.1. The purpose of staging is to separate those patients whose tumors are operable from those whose are not. The best chance of a long-term cure is the complete surgical resection of the tumor, but only 1 in 5 patients are operable at the time of presentation. The fact that almost 40% of patients who were considered to have operable T1 lesions are dead within five years suggests that staging needs to be improved.

TABLE 2.1. TNM Classification and Stage Grouping

DEFINITION OF TNM

Primary Tumor (T)

IX   Primary tumor cannot be assessed, or tumor proven by the presence of malignant cells in sputum or bronchial washings but not visualized by imaging or bronchoscopy

T0   No evidence of primary tumor

Tis Carcinoma *in situ*

T1   Tumor 3 cm or less in greatest dimension, surrounded by lung or visceral pleura, without bronchoscophic evidence of invasion more proximal than the lobar bronchus,* (i.e., not in the main bronchus)

T2   Tumor with any of the following features of size or extent:
More than 3 cm in greatest dimension
Involves main bronchus, 2 cm or more distal to the carina
Invades the visceral pleura
Associated with atelectasis or obstructive pneumonitis that extends to the hilar region but does not involve the entire lung

T3   Tumor of any size that directly invades any of the following: chest wall (including superior sulcus tumors), diaphragm, mediastinal pleura, parietal pericardium; or tumor in the main bronchus less than 2 cm distal to the carina, but without involvement of the carina; or associated atelectasis or obstructive pneumonitis of the entire lung

T4   Tumor of any size that invades any of the following: mediastinum, heart, great vessels, trachea, esophagus, vertebral body, carina; or separate tumor nodules in the same lobe; or tumor with malignant pleural effusion**

*Note: The uncommon superficial tumor of any size with its invasive component limited to the bronchial wall, which may extend proximal to the main bronchus, is also classified T1.

**Note: Most pleural effusions associated with lung cancer are due to tumor. However, there are a few patients in whom multiple cytopathologic examinations of pleural fluid are negative for tumor. In these cases, fluid is non-bloody and is not an exudate. Such patients may be further evaluated by videothoracoscopy (VATS) and direct pleural biopsies. When these elements and clinical judgment dictate that the effusion is not related to the tumor, the effusion should be excluded as a staging element and the patient should be staged T1, T2, or T3.

Regional Lymph Nodes (N)

NX   Regional lymph nodes cannot be assessed

N0   No regional lymph node metastasis

N1   Metastasis to ipsilateral peribronchial and/or ipsilateral hilar lymph nodes, and intrapulmonary nodes including involvement by direct extension of the primary tumor

TABLE 2.1. *Continued*

N2	Metastasis to ipsilateral mediastinal and/or subcarinal lymph nodes(s)		
N3	Metastasis to contralateral mediastinal, contralateral hilar, ipsilateral or contralateral scalene, or supraclavicular lymph nodes(s)		

Distant Metastasis (M)

MX   Distant metastasis cannot be assessed
M0   No distant metastasis
M1   Distant metastasis present

Note: M1 includes separate tumor nodule(s) in a different lobe (ipsilateral or contralateral).

STAGE GROUPING			
Occult Carcinoma	TX	N0	M0
Stage 0	Tis	N0	M0
Stage IA	T1	N0	M0
Stage IB	T2	N0	M0
Stage IIA	T1	N1	M0
Stage IIB	T2	N1	M0
	T3	N0	M0
Stage IIIA	T1	N2	M0
	T2	N2	M0
	T3	N1	M0
	T3	N2	M0
Stage IIIB	Any T	N3	M0
	T4	Any N	M0
Stage IV	Any T	Any N	M1

Source: Used with the permission of the American Joint Committee on Cancer (AJCC), Chicago, Illinois. The original source for this material is the AJCC Cancer Staging Manual, Sixth Edition (2002) published by Springer-New York, www.springeronline.com.

CASE 1

Figures 2.1 to 2.6 are images of a patient considered operable by conventional staging with contrast enhanced CT of the chest and upper abdomen. This patient has multiple soft tissue metastases only identified by the PET component of the study and not seen on CT.

Generally speaking, all patients with a diagnosis of small cell lung cancer are deemed inoperable, as this type represents a systemic disease process at the time of diagnosis. Still, treatment algorithms are changing, and some patients are considered for

FIGURE 2.1. Surgically resectable lung cancer using conventional staging.

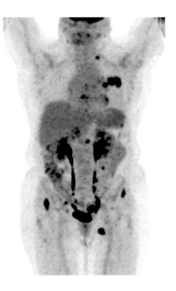

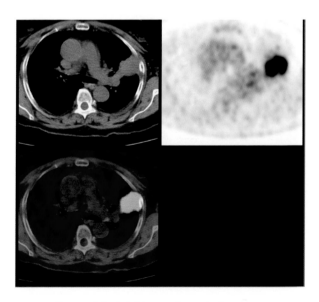

FIGURE 2.2. Axial image through the tumor.

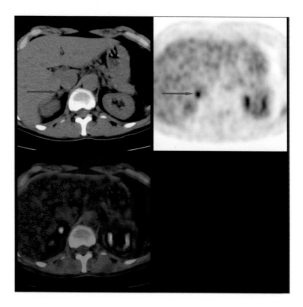

Figure 2.3. Metabolically active metastases in apparently normal right adrenal gland.

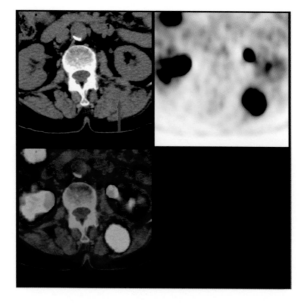

FIGURE 2.4. Soft tissue deposit in the left erector spinae muscle.

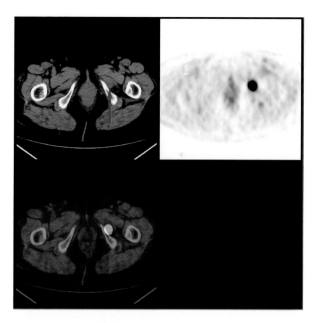

FIGURE 2.5. Unsuspected deposit in left obturator externus.

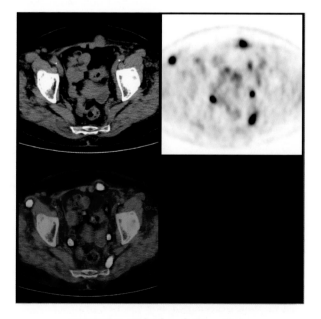

FIGURE 2.6. Multiple soft tissue Mets.

surgery and radiotherapy as part of their management of the disease. On the other hand, non-small cell lung cancer may be operable depending on conditions such as tumor site and size, as well as the presence or absence of distant metastatic involvement.

Surgery can be carried out with curative intent in those patients with limited stage disease, whereas palliative chemotherapy or radiotherapy is given to those considered inoperable. Stage IIIB and stage IV disease are considered inoperable, but controversy exists about the role of surgery in stage IIIA disease (with involved mediastinal nodes N2). Some patients who are considered unsuitable for surgery due to other comorbidity may be considered for radical radiotherapy.

To optimize patient outcome, it is necessary to obtain as much information as possible prior to deciding to follow a surgical pathway. It may be obvious from a plain chest X-ray that a tumor is inoperable. Features that make surgery unlikely include large tumors extending across the midline, bilateral lesions, malignant effusions, enlarged mediastinal nodes, or any evidence of pulmonary or osseous metastases.

Over the last 20 years there has been a rapid growth in the use of functional metabolic imaging in the diagnosis of lung cancer. Initially this was in the form of PET only but recently this has been superseded by the advent of fused PET/CT technology. The use of PET and PET/CT has primarily been in the characterization of the solitary pulmonary nodule (SPN) and the preoperative staging of non-small cell lung cancer (NSCLC). Recently other applications for its utilization have been found in detecting recurrence and in the evolving fields of radiotherapy planning and assessment of treatment response.

The Role of PET/CT in Lung Cancer
Assessment of the solitary pulmonary nodule (SPN)
Staging of non-small cell lung cancer (NSCLC)
Assessment of mediastinal lymphadenopathy
Identification of distant metastatic disease
Detection of recurrent disease

With increasing evidence of its use in the following:
Radiotherapy planning
Response to therapy assessment
As a prognostic indicator
? Role in staging small cell lung cancer

SOLITARY PULMONARY NODULES

Soliary pulmonary nodules occur in about 1 in 500 chest X-rays and approximately half are malignant in nature. The assessment of such nodules has proved difficult using conventional imaging with CT. Nodules that are seen to contain fat or calcification on the CT scan are felt more likely to be benign and rapidly growing lesions with spiculated margins are considered more sinister.

Despite detailed CT analysis many lesions are still classified as indeterminate following assessment. These indeterminate cases require further evaluation with a histological tissue sample from the nodule. If the clinical and radiological features are reassuring, a watch-and-wait policy may be taken, with regular scanning to assess any interval change. There has been a wide variation in the sensitivity and specificity of both bronchoscopy and transthoracic needle biopsy in the detection of malignancy in these indeterminate cases.

It is clear that conventional imaging and attempts to obtain histology of small pulmonary nodules is a difficult and often unrewarding exercise. PET/CT has high sensitivity, specificity, and accuracy in the characterization of solitary pulmonary nodules. Many articles have been published with a generally accepted mean sensitivity of about 96%, a lower specificity of 78% and a diagnostic accuracy of over 92%.

In general the increased uptake within a pulmonary nodule can be assessed in two ways, either visually, by comparing the intensity of the nodule with the background bloodpool activity or by means of an SUV measurement. The SUV uses a suggested cut-off value of approximately 2.5 to discriminate between benign and malignant processes. There is evidence to suggest that both methods are of similar accuracy in the determination of abnormal increased activity.

What has become clear over the course of the past few years is that not all metabolically active nodules are malignant and indeed an arbitrary cut off value of 2.5 cannot be regarded as wholly accurate. Benign lesions can occasionally have quite intense uptake and some malignant lesions may be quite quiescent. Of note some carcinoid and neuroendocrine lesions have been reported as being causes of false negative studies. In addition, scar adenocarcinomas and bronchoalveolar carcinomas can be difficult to detect. In our experience however these lesions often do show low grade but abnormal uptake.

The most common benign causes are granulomatous conditions, such as TB, histoplasmosis or coccidiomycosis. Sarcoidosis can also be the cause of uptake within nodules as can active

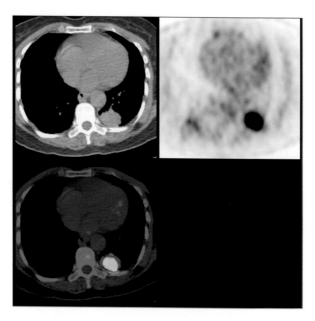

FIGURE 2.7. Metabolically active pulmonary nodule.

inflammatory processes although these conditions often have characteristic scan patterns.

Other causes of false-positive scans include adenomas, hamartomas, neurofibromas and fibrosis. Figure 2.7 shows a left-sided pulmonary nodule. The PET component of the study is positive, and the histological diagnosis was NSCLC. Figures 2.8

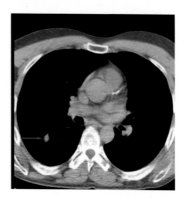

FIGURE 2.8. Solitary pulmonary nodule. Benign or malignant?

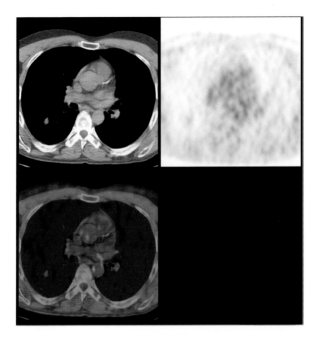

FIGURE 2.9. No activity. Diagnosis: benign bronchocoele.

and 2.9. show a 1.5 cm right SPN. The PET scan was negative and the diagnosis was a benign bronchocele that is resolved with conservative treatment and physiotherapy. Figures 2.10 and 2.11 illustrate bilateral pulmonary nodules showing FDG uptake. The histological diagnosis is pulmonary sarcoidosis.

Top Tip
Approximately 85% of metabolically active pulmonary nodules are malignant. If an FDG positive pulmonary nodule is found, it should be assumed to be malignant until proved otherwise.

The principle causes of false negative scans are lesions that are too small (less than 1 cm) for accurate resolution by the PET camera or well-differentiated malignant lesions with little or no FDG uptake. The advent of fused PET/CT imaging has resulted in

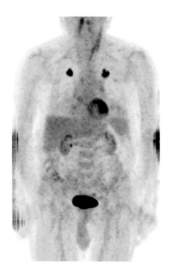

FIGURE 2.10. Bilateral pulmonary nodules. Diagnosis: metabolically active pulmonary sarcoidosis.

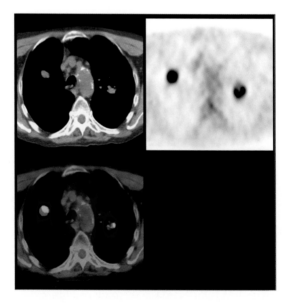

FIGURE 2.11. Bilateral pulmonary nodules. Diagnosis: metabolically active pulmonary sarcoidosis.

an improvement in reporting confidence, and early anecdotal evidence suggests increased lesion detection. Small lesions with poor uptake not seen on the PET component of the study may be detected on the CT component when viewed in lung windows. Lesions as small as 1 mm to 2 mm can be detected in this way and, although they are too small for accurate characterization by CT, their presence can be identified and monitored with serial imaging. In this patient group, it is suspected that the nodules have a slower rate of growth and are better differentiated, because a lower SUV is associated with longer tumor doubling times and decreased DNA proliferation rates. Therefore a delay in diagnosis may not be as significant within this particular patient group.

False Positive SPN	False Negative SPN
Granulomatous conditions	Bronchoalveolar cancer
Sarcoidosis	Scar adenocarinoma
Inflammation	Carcinoid tumors
Infection	Neuroendocrine tumors
Adenomas	
Hamartomas	but primarily....
Neurofibromas	Lesions that are too small (<1 cm)
Pulmonary fibrosis	Well-differentiated lesions

STAGING OF NON-SMALL CELL LUNG CANCER
In making the decision to proceed to surgery all relevant information should be gathered. At present conventional staging will use a combination of contrast enhanced CT of the chest and upper abdomen (to include the adrenal glands and liver-both common sites of metastatic disease), mediastinoscopy, transbronchial needle biopsy and even MRI.

CASE 2
Figures 2.12 and 2.13 are the MIP and axial images through a left upper lobe pulmonary mass. The mass has a homogenous appearance on the CT scan but only the periphery of the lesion shows FDG uptake on the PET component. This appearance is commonly seen with active peripheral tumor and central necrosis. The initial histology was undiagnostic because the edge of

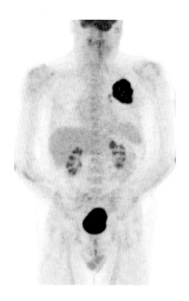

FIGURE 2.12. Cavitating pulmonary mass. Initial histology undiagnositic.

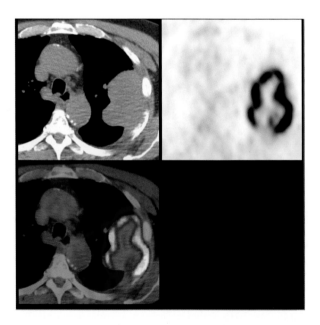

FIGURE 2.13. Cavitating pulmonary mass. Initial histology undiagnostic.

the lesion was not sampled. Repeat biopsy following the PET/CT scan revealed a diagnosis of squamous cell cancer (which often cavitates).

CT is a satisfactory method for the assessment of the size and location of a primary pulmonary lesion, but it is less successful in the characterization of mediastinal nodes. In general radiological practice mediastinal nodes greater than 1 cm in diameter are considered abnormal and therefore more likely to represent metastatic disease. Unfortunately the accuracy of such a system is only approximately 60% to 79%, as small nodes may contain malignant cells and large nodes are often only reactive in nature, CT can therefore under or overstage up to 40% of cases. Studies have shown that up to 75% of metastatic nodes were within nodes considered to be of normal size. Using a smaller size as the cut off for normal nodes has not been shown to improve sensitivity and, in fact, results in a decrease in both specificity and overall accuracy.

The use of mediastinoscopy has been reserved for those patients considered suitable for surgery by CT staging but who have enlarged mediastinal nodes that require evaluation. This procedure is not without its risks and may have a false negative rate of up to 10%. Although transbronchial needle biopsy can have a very high specificity it has a poor sensitivity of not much more than 50%, and in turn can have a significant morbidity. Several large retrospective and prospective trials have established the superiority of PET over CT in the staging of mediastinal lymph nodes. The conclusion of many studies being that nodal size is a poor determinant of metastatic involvement. Arita et al examined lymph nodes of all sizes, in known lung cancer patients and found that, in those nodes with metastatic deposits the nodal size was "normal" in 74%.

Figure 2.14 shows enlarged reactive axillary and mediastinal nodes, but no abnormal metabolic activity. Figure 2.15 shows a small FDG avid mediastinal node. The mediastinoscopy revealed metastatic adenocarcinoma.

Top Tip
The conventional staging of nodes by size criteria alone can often lead to the wrong conclusion. Metabolic imaging stages mediastinal nodes with much greater accuracy than CT alone.

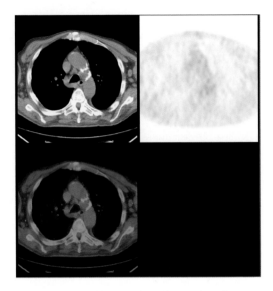

FIGURE 2.14. Enlarged axillary and mediastinal nodes. Reactive only without FDG uptake.

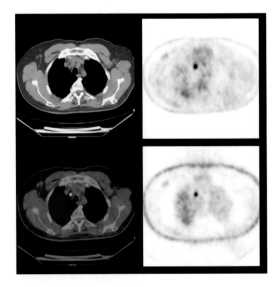

FIGURE 2.15. Small active mediastinal node. Metastatic adenocarcinoma cell found following mediastinoscopy.

FIGURE 2.16. MIP image showing a
left hilar lesion.

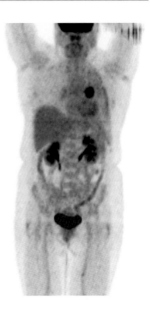

The highest diagnostic accuracy has been with combined
PET/CT with a generally accepted figure of approximately 90%
for mediastinal nodal involvement. In particular, PET has
consistently been shown to be accurate in the distinction
between N2 (operable) and N3 (inoperable) nodal disease.
Figures 2.16 and 2,17 are MIP and axial views that demonstrate
a left hilar primary tumor with distal collapse of the left upper
lobe and an inactive left pleural effusion.

Top Tip
Without the aid of PET/CT it can be difficult to distin-
guish active tumor from collapsed lung or necrotic tissue.
See Figures 2.12, 2.13, 2.17, 2.32, and 2.33.

Pieterman prospectively compared standard contrast enhanced CT staging of the mediastinum to PET prior to surgical
resection and found that not only was PET approximately 20%
more sensitive and specific than CT, but PET also identified
unknown distant metastatic disease in 10% of cases. Since a negative PET scan has such a high predictive value, the patient may
proceed to surgery without any further staging.

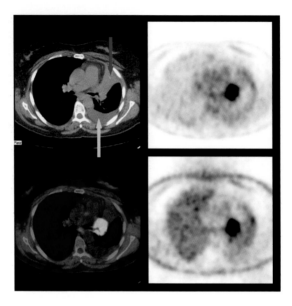

FIGURE 2.17. MIP image showing a left hilar lesion with associated inactive left upper lobe collapse (red arrow) and pleural effusion (yellow arrow).

Not only is PET/CT superior than other noninvasive methods for mediastinal staging, it also has the advantage that whole body images are obtainable and therefore an assessment can be made of potential distant metastatic disease. A wide range of reports have demonstrated the effectiveness of PET and PET/CT in the detection of unsuspected distant metastatic disease, with unsuspected disease identified in 11% to 44% of cases. Several studies have shown metabolic imaging to be more accurate than combined conventional imaging consisting of a contrast enhanced CT scan of chest and abdomen in combination with bone scanning.

The common sites of metastases from NSCLC are to the adrenal glands, liver, bone, and brain. PET and PET/CT are accurate in the assessment of metastatic disease to the liver and adrenal glands. Despite reports to the contrary it is our experience that many of the detected adrenal metastases are within morphologically normal adrenal glands, however this may reflect the fact that we use PET/CT for the preoperative staging of all pulmonary masses.

In general, lytic osseous metatases appear to have a greater uptake of FDG and as such are more readily detected. In fact evidence exists to suggest that PET may be less sensitive than bone scanning for osteoblastic metastases but other reports suggest that PET/CT is both more sensitive and specific than bone scanning in lesion detection in lung cancer.

EXAMPLES OF UNSUSPECTED DISEASE FOLLOWING CONVENTIONAL STAGING

Figures 2.18 and 2.19 show a right hilar tumor with an undiagnosed metastatic deposit in the right adrenal gland. Both the right and left adrenal glands are morphologically normal, so no CT abnormality was identified.

> **Top Tip**
> Evidence suggests that the removal of a solitary adrenal deposit at the time of resection of the lung primary results in an increased life expectancy.
> Liver, adrenal, brain and bony deposits are common with lung cancer but many of the lesions are undetected in the course of conventional staging.

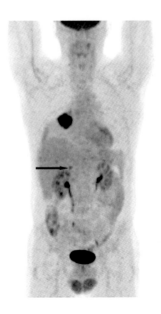

FIGURE 2.18. Right hilar mass with unsuspected right adrenal metastases.

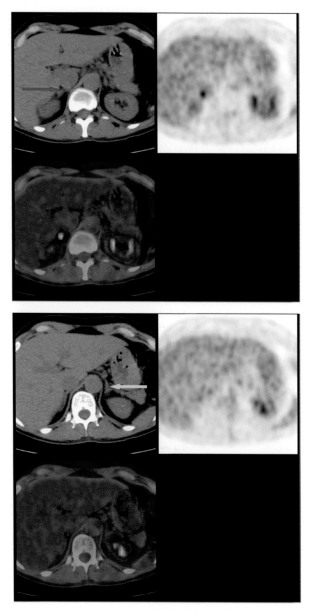

FIGURE 2.19. Normal left adrenal and unsuspected metastatic deposit in right adrenal.

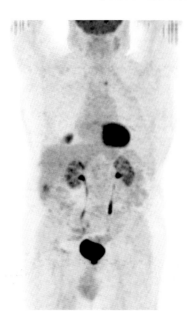

FIGURE 2.20. Right lung primary with liver secondary deposit.

Figures 2.20 to 2.22 show a right lower lobe non-small cell lung cancer with a subcapsular deposit to the right lobe of liver. Figures 2.23 to 2.25 show a right lung tumor with involved right hilar nodes and an isolated left gluteal metastatic deposit.

Top Tip
The background activated brown fat uptake complicates interpretation of the PET study but the brown fat can clearly be distinguished from nodal deposition on the CT component of the study.

Figures 2.26 to 2.28 are examples of bony deposits only found on PET/CT. No CT abnormality demonstrated. None of these lesions

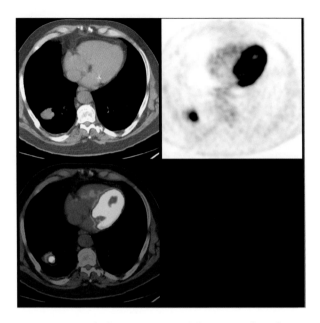

FIGURE 2.21. Right lung primary with liver secondary deposit.

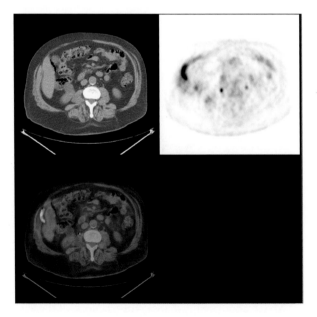

FIGURE 2.22. Right lung primary with liver secondary deposit.

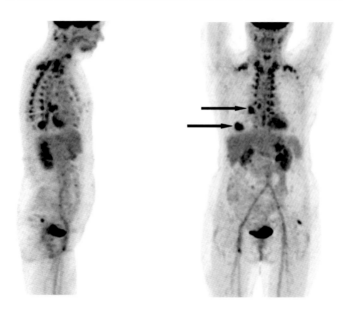

FIGURE 2.23. AP and lateral MIP views. Right lung primary with right hilar nodes and marked brown fat uptake in the neck and thorax.

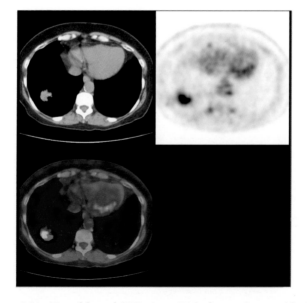

FIGURE 2.24. AP and lateral MIP views. Right lung primary with right hilar nodes and marked brown fat uptake in the neck and thorax.

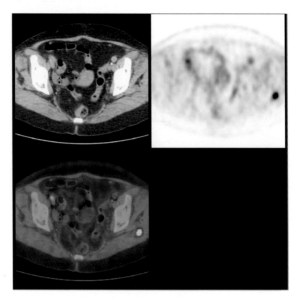

FIGURE 2.25. An isolated left gluteal deposit confirmed metastatic non-small cell lung cancer.

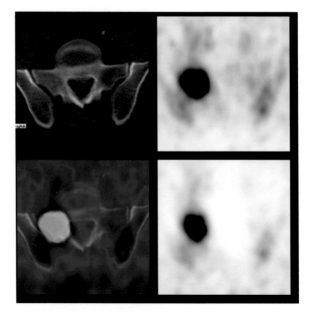

FIGURE 2.26. Deposit in right sacral ala.

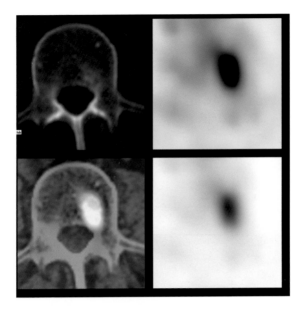

FIGURE 2.27. Deposit in vertebral body.

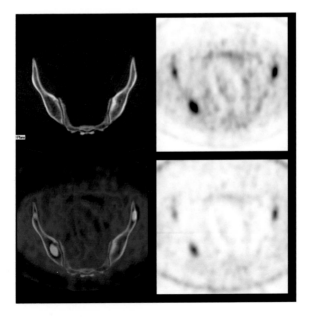

FIGURE 2.28. Deposits in both iliac wings.

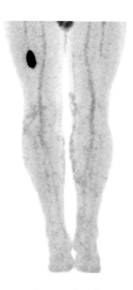

FIGURE 2.29. Unsuspected right femoral shaft deposit from lung primary.

were detected on bone scanning either. Figures 2.29 to 2.31 illustrate a right mid-femoral secondary deposit from a lung primary. Notice the subtle thinning and expansion of the bony

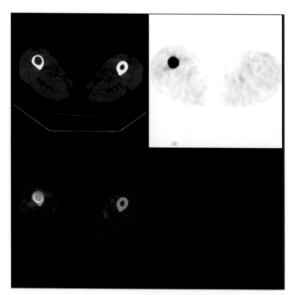

FIGURE 2.30. Unsuspected right femoral shaft deposit from lung primary DT.

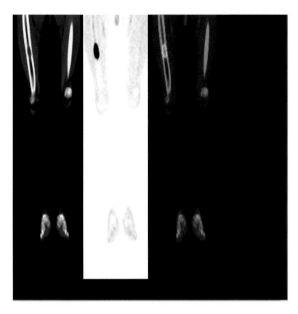

FIGURE 2.31. Unsuspected right femoral shaft deposit from lung primary DT.

cortex. Conventional CT staging would not extend below the liver and adrenal glands and therefore this lesion would not be seen.

DETECTION OF RECURRENT DISEASE

The detection of recurrent disease can be hampered by the confounding effects of either radiotherapy or postoperative inflammatory change. If radiotherapy has been given, a post therapy radiation pneumonitis can occur, and although this may have a characteristic appearance on the CT component of the study, it may be difficult to exclude recurrent disease. In these cases it is recommended that a PET/CT scan should not be carried out any less than three months after the therapy to allow any metabolically active macrophage activity within inflammatory lung to resolve preventing a false-positive report. A similar time scale is suggested to allow postoperative change to improve. The primary purpose of staging is to allow informed decisions to take place as to the most appropriate therapy for the patient. Several studies have clearly shown that TMN stage, as indicated by PET/CT, relates to the overall survival figures in an approximately linear fashion, whereas the staging with CT alone does not. In addition to the more accurate staging, PET/CT also acts as an independent prognostic indicator. Many studies have been carried out assessing the FDG activity of the primary tumor and relating this to overall survival figures. Ahuja and coworkers showed that those patients with an SUV greater than 10 had a median survival of less than those with SUV less than 10. Dhital found a median survival of less than 6 months when the SUV was in excess of 20. The converse has also been shown to be true, tumors with lower grade activity of SUV less than 5 have (and stage I disease clinically) have more than five times the five year survival rate compared with those having an SUV greater than five.

It has further been shown that the FDG uptake correlates with both the tumor growth and proliferation rates as well as the degree of tumor differention. Most prognostic information so far obtained relates to non small cell lung cancer but scant research has indicated that the SUV may also provide prognostic information for small cell cancer.

PET/CT IN THERAPY RESPONSE AND RADIOTHERAPY PLANNING

As we have already shown the FDG uptake relates well to tumor growth and proliferation rates. This allows us to quantify the metabolic response of therapy within the tumor. Weber and his coworkers found that a decline of SUV of more than 20% following therapy correlated well with the overall response to therapy. The response also correlated with the mean time to progression and overall survival. Debate exists as to the most appropriate time to carry out a response scan. Results as early as one week after initiation of chemotherapy accurately reflect response but imaging six weeks after chemotherapy has finished and at least three months after radiotherapy is generally regarded as more accurate. This helps avoid the problems with false positive reports due to radiation induced pneumonitis.

It has also been shown that those tumors with higher pretherapy FDG uptake respond better to radiotherapy than those with low uptake and additionally persisting uptake after therapy was predictive of relapse.

Recent work has been carried out to investigate the use of PET/CT in radiotherapy planning. It is obviously important to have adequate coverage of the tumor volume but to avoid unnecessary irradiation of normal tissues. PET/CT has been shown to be better than CT at assessing accurate tumor volume. In par-

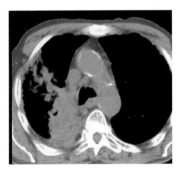

FIGURE 2.32. Patient for radiotherapy. Where does the tumor end and the collapsed lung begin?

ticular PET/CT is excellent at delineating tumor from distal atelectasis.

Figure 2.32 shows an example of a central tumor with distal collapse, the margins of which can not be clearly separated on CT alone. Figure 2.33 is the fused PET/CT image and it clearly shows the central active tumor and the distal collapsed lung allowing a limited radiation port and thus sparing normal tissues.

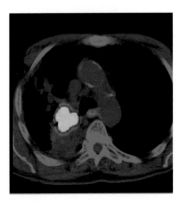

FIGURE 2.33. Patient for radiotherapy. Where does the tumor end and the collapsed lung begin?

SMALL CELL LUNG CANCER AND MESOTHELIOMA

It had previously been accepted that a diagnosis of small cell lung cancer equates to a diagnosis of disseminated disease. This, however, is not always the case. Rarely, a localized small cell cancer is found that can be surgically resected with curative intent or treated with combined chemoradiotherapy. Generally the principle role of staging in small cell lung cancer is to determine if localized radiotherapy can be used in addition to chemotherapy.

The role of PET/CT in this instance is still under evaluation but evidence suggests PET can be used to accurately upstage presumed limited disease and has been shown to be useful in the detection of paraneoplastic associated small cell lung cancers. PET/CT has been shown to be sensitive in the detection of mesothelioma, often found in active pleural plaques in patients previously exposed to asbestos.

Figures 2.34 and 2.35 show AP and lateral MIP views of a young female patient diagnosed with mesothelioma. Notice the

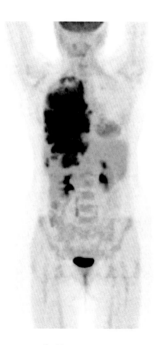

FIGURE 2.34. Right lung mesothelioma. No previous asbestos exposure.

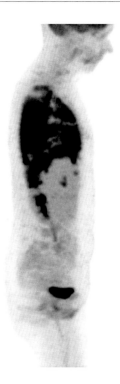

FIGURE 2.35. Right lung mesothelioma. No previous asbestos exposure.

circumferential pleural uptake of FDG which is characteristic of this disease. Figure 2.36 illustrates an axial view through the thickened metabolically active pleura in the same patient. Figure 2.37 demonstrates the appearance of normal vocal cord uptake due to the patient talking during the uptake period post injection of FDG. Figure 2.38 shows asymmetric uptake of FDG within the right but not the left vocal cord. This appearance could be caused by a malignancy of the right vocal cord but in this case the right cord is normal. We are seeing normal uptake in the right cord and decreased uptake in the left as a result of a left recurrent laryngeal nerve palsy from a left hilar mass.

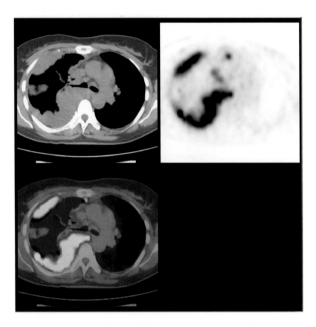

FIGURE 2.36. Right lung mesothelioma. No previous asbestos exposure. Axial view showing the thickened pleura.

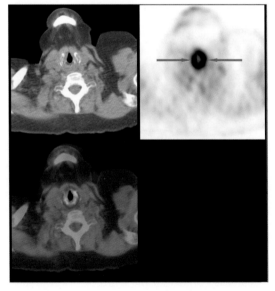

FIGURE 2.37. Symmetric vocal cord uptake as a result of talking after injection of FDG.

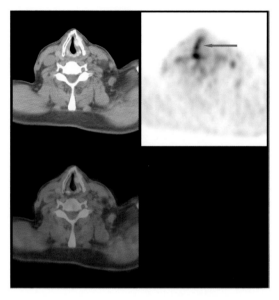

FIGURE 2.38. Decreased vocal cord uptake on the left as a result of left recurrent laryngeal nerve palsy from a left hilar tumor.

Chapter 3

Lymphoma

INTRODUCTION

Lymphoma is generally divided into two groups: Hodgkin's disease (HD) and an inhomogeneous group of conditions called non-Hodgkin's lymphoma (NHL). HD tends to involve a single nodal group and spread in a fixed pattern along the lymphatic chain. NHL is a multifocal disease which often presents late with disseminated spread.

Lymphoma tends to be both chemosensitive and radiosensitive. Localized disease can be effectively treated with radiotherapy, but disseminated spread requires systemic chemotherapy.

	Hodgkin's Disease	Non-Hodgkin's
Incidence	3 per 10,000	20 per 10,000
Peak age	Bimodal 20–30y and >70y	Increases with age Most >40y
Male:Female	3M:2F	8M:7F
Spread	Orderly progression along lymph chains	Less orderly, often multifocal
5-year survival	70–80%	40–70%
Treatment	Localized-radiotherapy Disseminated-chemotherapy	Localized-radiotherapy Disseminated- chemotherapy

The prognosis of a patient with lymphoma is related to the disease stage at presentation. Accurate, effective staging is required to guide the appropriate therapeutic pathway. The Ann Arbor classification (Table 3.1) is commonly used for the staging of lymphomas. Originally developed for Hodgkin's disease, this staging scheme was later expanded to include non-Hodgkin's lymphoma.

TABLE 3.1. Staging of Lymphoma: Ann Arbor Classification

Stage I
Involvement of a single lymph node region (I) or of a single
extralymphatic organ or site (IE)

Stage II
Involvement of two or more lymph node regions on the same side of
the diaphragm (II) or localized involvement of extra-lymphatic organ
or site and of one or more lymph node regions on the same side of the
diaphragm (IIE).

Stage III
Involvement of lymph node regions on both sides of the diaphragm
(III) which may also be accompanied by localized involvement of
extralymphatic organ or site (IIIE) or by involvement of the spleen
(IIIS) or both (IIISE)

Stage IV
Diffuse or disseminated involvement of one or more extralymphatic
organs or tissues with or without associated lymph node enlargement

Source: Lister TA, Crowther D, Sutcliffe SB, et al. Report of a committee
convened to discuss the evaluation and staging of patients with Hodgkin's
disease. *J Clin Oncol* 1989;7:1630–1636.

Over the last 10 to 15 years, PET scanning has emerged as a
powerful imaging modality in the assessment of patients with
both Hodgkin's and non-Hodgkin's lymphoma. PET/CT is not
only used to identify sites of residual disease after therapy but is
a useful tool in staging, restaging, identifying potential biopsy
sites and quantifying the response to therapy. Since a PET/CT
scan can be used to image the whole body it gives an accurate
anatomical distribution of the disease burden within the patient,
allowing the appropriate therapeutic pathway to be chosen.

The Role of PET/CT in Lymphoma
- Assess response to therapy/residual disease
- Identify recurrent disease
- Initial diagnosis and staging
- Identify suitable sites for biopsy

and possibly

- Disease surveillance
- Radiotherapy planning

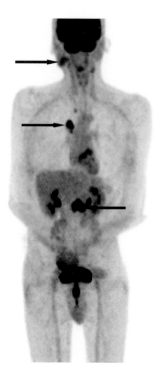

FIGURE 3.1. An example of stage 4 disease. NHL with disease in the mediastinum, neck, and abdomen.

Figure 3.1 is an example of a patient with known non-Hodgkin's lymphoma within right sided neck nodes. After the PET/CT scan this patient was upstaged from stage I to stage IV disease. Active disease was found in the neck, mediastinum and abdomen as indicated by the arrows. Normal uptake and excretion is seen in the brain and urinary system respectively.

ASSESSMENT OF TREATMENT RESPONSE

There is increasing evidence that PET/CT scans carried out after two cycles of chemotherapy are predictive of disease-free survival and overall survival rate. Those patients with a PET positive scan after therapy are at high risk of recurrent disease and further, more aggressive, therapy should be considered. If the posttherapy PET scan does not show abnormal uptake, the prognosis is better, but some of these patients relapse in due course. Recent research suggests that the tumor marker bcl2 is related to that group of tumors that initially respond to therapy but later relapse. Further research is required to determine if this subgroup would benefit from continued PET surveillance.

Case I

This is a 40-year-old male who presented with night sweats, an enlarged spleen, and palpable neck nodes. Biopsy confirmed a diagnosis of diffuse large B-cell lymphoma. A pretherapy PET/CT scan revealed extensive disease both above and below the diaphragm. Metabolically active disease is seen in the neck, mediastinum, left axilla, and spleen, and extending along both the paraaortic and aortocaval nodes. He was treated with chemotherapy and a post therapy PET/CT scan revealed a complete metabolic response to therapy.

Figure 3.2 is the pretherapy MIP (maximum intensity projection image) showing active disease in the left side of the neck and left axilla. Further disease is seen in the mediastinum and spleen. Both the aorto-caval and para-aortic nodal chains are involved. Figure 3.3 compares the pretherapy and posttherapy studies. After therapy, it reveals only normal physiological FDG uptake within the brain, heart, liver and spleen. Normal excretion of FDG is identified in the kidneys ureters and bladder. The patient remained disease free at two years posttherapy.

The assessment of treatment response following the administration of chemotherapy is a relatively new and exciting area in which PET/CT is leading all other imaging modalities. Since lymphomas are by and large chemo- and radiosensitive, a rapid

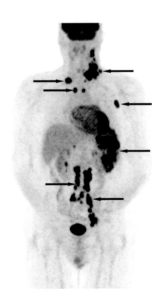

FIGURE 3.2. Pretherapy MIP.

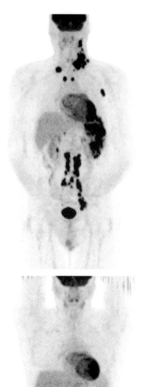

FIGURE 3.3. Pretherapy and posttherapy studies showing a complete metabolic response to therapy.

change in their glycolytic pattern is seen following successful therapy. Figure 3.4 compares pretherapy and posttherapy MIP images in a patient with a gastric lymphoma. Again, the activity within the tumor has switched off completely, which is a good prognostic indicator.

An FDG-PET scan early in the chemotherapy regime can provide an accurate classification of patients and differentiate responders from nonresponders. No consensus has universally established how soon after therapy one should carry out a

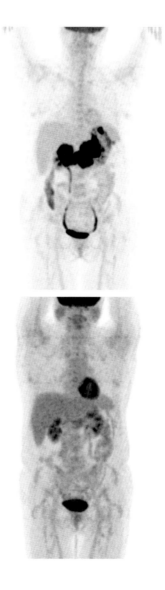

FIGURE 3.4. Pretherapy and post-therapy scans in a case of gastric lymphoma. This is the complete response to therapy.

PET/CT scan, but both false positive and false negative results do occur if scanning is carried out too soon.

PET/CT IN RECURRENT DISEASE

PET/CT has been shown to be the most effective tool in the assessment of recurrent lymphoma and has a higher sensitivity and specificity than CT and MRI combined.

Case 2

This case shows a patient with a previous history of a high-grade esophageal lymphoma. A left axillary node was palpable on routine examination. CT scan demonstrated a 3 cm left axillary node and some small paraaortic nodes which were felt to be insignificant as they had not changed significantly from a previous CT scan. The patient underwent a PET/CT scan to help characterize the axillary node and assess for further disease. Figures 3.5 to 3.8 show the MIP (5) and selected axial images revealing active axillary (6), paraaortic (7) and external iliac nodes (8). The PET/CT scan revealed active left axillary, paraaortic, and left external iliac nodes, thereby demonstrating a more extensive recurrence than had been suspected.

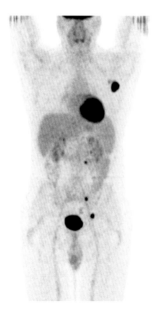

FIGURE 3.5. Recurrence of high-grade esophageal lymphoma.

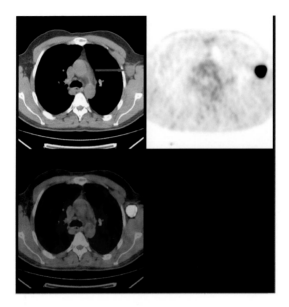

FIGURE 3.6. Left axillary node.

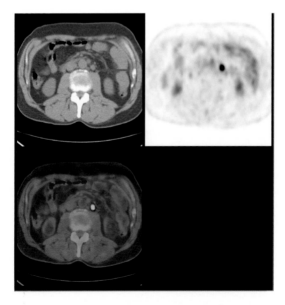

FIGURE 3.7. Active paraaortic node.

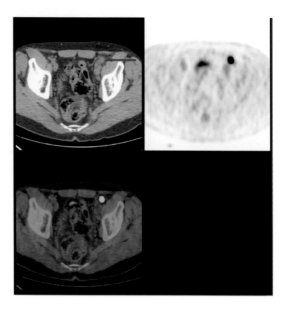

FIGURE 3.8. Active left external iliac node.

Case 3

This is middle-aged male with a possible recurrence of high-grade T-cell lymphoma. He re-presented with abdominal pain and night sweats. Normal CT scan of chest, abdomen and pelvis. Figure 3.9 is an MIP view that demonstrates two areas of abnormal uptake. The first in the right lower abdomen and the second at the right lung hilum. Figures 3.10 and 3.11 show the focal uptake as it relates to a small bowel recurrence in the distal ileum and a further involved node at the right hilum. Both these lesions were confirmed histologically.

Top Tip
These patients could have proceeded to local radiotherapy for an assumed solitary site of recurrence. PET/CT upstaged the disease and appropriate systemic treatment was administered.

FIGURE 3.9. Possible recurrence of high-grade T-cell lymphoma.

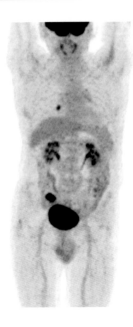

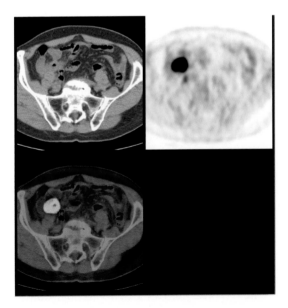

FIGURE 3.10. Possible recurrence of high-grade T-cell lymphoma. Note the abnormal focal uptake of FDG in the distal small bowel. No abnormality was detected on the CT.

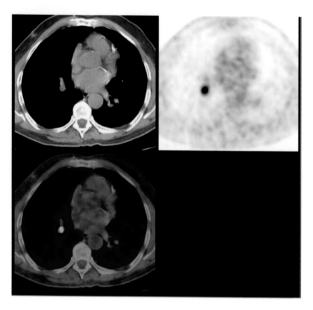

FIGURE 3.11. Unsuspected abnormal focus of FDG uptake at the right lung hilum.

POSTTHERAPY RESIDUAL MASSES

Conventional imaging with CT is often used to assess the patient after completion of therapy. The CT scan can not accurately differentiate between a posttherapy fibrotic mass and an area of residual active disease. Because the PET component of the scan assesses metabolic activity rather than anatomy, residual disease can be identified. A complete metabolic response to therapy correlates well with patient long-term outcome. However those patients with abnormal FDG uptake following therapy are at high risk of recurrent disease (>90%) and more aggressive therapy should be considered. Debate exists about the most suitable time to perform a post therapy PET/CT but scans carried out after only two or three cycles of chemotherapy are predictive of disease free and overall survival rates.

Case 4

A 55-year-old male with a history of treated follicular NHL. The patient had a PET/CT scan 6 weeks after chemotherapy to assess the metabolic response to treatment. You should study carefully the posttherapy image in Figure 3.12 and try to identify any sites of abnormal uptake. The arrows in Figure 3.12a identify the

FIGURE 3.12. Posttherapy residual
abnormal uptake.

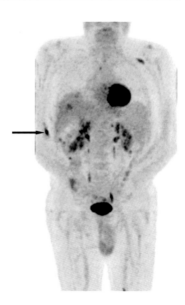

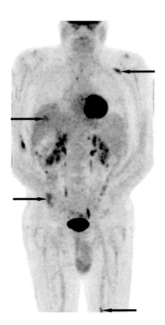

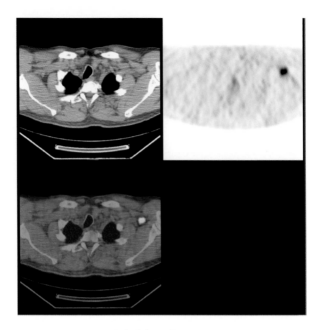

FIGURE 3.13. Subtle left axillary node missed on CT.

sites of residual disease. Did you spot the small focus of disease in the medial aspect of the left thigh? On this occasion, there has not been a complete response to therapy and residual uptake is seen in the left axilla, liver, and right hemipelvis. A further subtle focus of FDG uptake is found within the muscles of the medial left thigh.

Figures 3.13 to 3.16 demonstrate the subtle findings missed by CT in the same patient. The patient went on to have more aggressive therapy but failed to respond and died 18 months after this PET/CT scan. These images clearly show how effective PET/CT can be when compared with conventional CT assessment of therapeutic response.

Top Tip
Posttherapy PET/CT assessment identifies residual disease more accurately than any other modality.

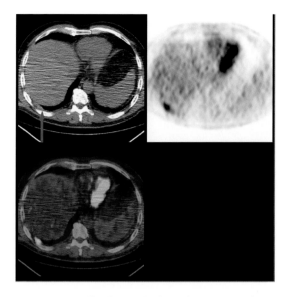

FIGURE 3.14. Small subcapsular liver deposit missed on CT.

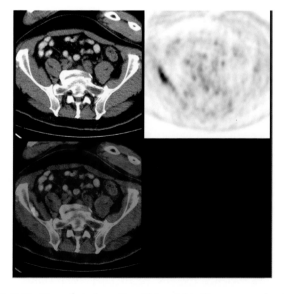

FIGURE 3.15. Muscular deposit within right iliacus muscle deposit missed on CT.

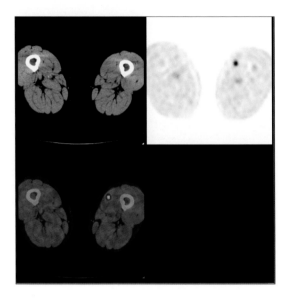

FIGURE 3.16. Another example of a muscular deposit within the right iliacus muscle. This lesion was not detected on CT.

INITIAL DIAGNOSIS AND STAGING

PET/CT has a high sensitivity (>90%) for the detection of most of the common types of lymphoma. It is less reliable with MALT lymphoma and small lymphocytic NHL of which between 50 and 90% are reportedly detected by PET.

It is important remember that false-positive uptake can sometimes be seen in inflammatory and granulomatous conditions as a result of macrophage activity. The macrophages utilize considerable energy during respiratory bursts as they digest unwanted debris around inflamed tissue. This is why histological confirmation is required when abnormal uptake is detected. In this regard a staging PET/CT can demonstrate the distribution of disease burden and also identify suitable candidate sites for biopsy.

The staging system for lymphoma has been outlined earlier. Staging can identify those patients who would benefit from localized or extended field radiotherapy and differentiate the group that require systemic therapy. PET/CT has been shown to stage lymphoma more accurately than CT scanning, gallium scintigraphy or PET alone.

FIGURE 3.17. Unusual presentation of follicular lymphoma of the scalp.

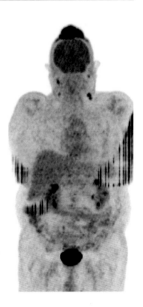

Case 5
An unusual presentation of follicular lymphoma of the scalp. This patient had a histologically confirmed follicular lymphoma but conventional imaging had only revealed small nodes in the neck. These nodes were considered to be within normal limits. PET/CT scan was used to assess these nodes and show if there was evidence of any distant disease. Figure 3.17 is the MIP image, the streaky black vertical lines are due to artifact, a feature often seen when scanning larger patients.

The PET/CT scan demonstrated uptake in small neck nodes bilaterally. These nodes were biopsied under ultrasound guideance and found to contain follicular lymphoma. These nodes are demonstrated on the axial images presented in Figure 3.18.

Top Tip
The PET/CT scan findings can be used to find candidate nodes for histological sampling. There are more than 300 nodes found within the head and neck in any normal individual and size criteria is not a good discriminator on which to base possible tumoral involvement.

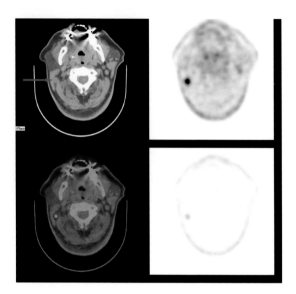

FIGURE 3.18. Small involved right-sided neck nodes.

PRETRANSPLANT ASSESSMENT

Studies have been carried out to assess the effectiveness of FDG-PET in comparison to CT in those patients with aggressive lymphomas (both NHL and HD) who were undergoing salvage cytoreductive chemotherapy followed by high-dose chemotherapy and autologous stem cell transplantation. Results have shown that the PET findings correlate strongly with disease free survival and can be used to predict the post transplant outcome with high accuracy. The predictive accuracy of PET was more than 90% compared to less than 60% for CT.

PEDIATRICS

Although the data supporting the use of FDG PET in pediatric lymphoma is much less than that for adult patients, early data suggest that [18]FDG PET is as valuable in this age group as with adults.

A retrospective study of pediatric tumors, including 60 patients with Hodgkin's and non-Hodgkin's lymphoma, found that PET was helpful in 75% of cases and altered management in 32%. In a further study, compared to CT, FDG PET led to different staging in 6 out of 25 pediatric mixed lymphoma cases (4 upstaged, 2 downstaged). Another retrospective study of Hodgkin's and non-Hodgkin's lymphoma showed that FDG PET changed disease stage and treatment in 10.5% of patients at initial staging, correctly evaluated early response in 16 of 19 patients, showed a specificity of 95% in patients at the end of treatment and a specificity of 94% in systematic follow up (compared to 54% and 66% with conventional methods respectively).

A difference between assessment the of adults and children in lymphoma is the increased frequency of thymic activity in the latter. While normal thymic activity can usually be recognized, it can occasionally cause difficulty in interpretation in children with residual anterior mediastinal masses following treatment.

PET/CT AS A PROGNOSTIC TOOL
The intensity of uptake and its relation to mitotic index, tumor differentiation, and long-term prognosis is not clearly defined and remains the subject of debate. It is fair to say that the response to therapy, comparing pretherapy and posttherapy scans, can provide an indication to long-term outcome. An international prognostic index of lymphoma exists and includes information such as age, sex, tumor stage, and serum markers. Whether PET/CT will eventually be included as a prognostic indicator remains to be seen.

TUMOR SURVEILLANCE
Recurrence of disease is common with both HD and NHL. Effective treatments exist for recurrent Hodgkin's disease that can stimulate remission or cure. The more advanced the stage, the poorer the prognosis.

Unfortunately low-grade NHL proves ultimately fatal in most patients. Long periods of remission are possible with appropriate therapy and cure is possible in some cases. The cure rate for high grade lymphoma usually lies in the range of 50 to 70%. Early detection of recurrence is essential to maximize the impact of therapy. Delayed diagnosis, particularly in Hodgkin's may result in increased mortality.

A posttherapy PET/CT scan with abnormal uptake necessitates further more aggressive therapy for that patient (assuming reactive or inflammatory uptake is outruled). A normal posttherapy PET/CT presents a more difficult dilemma. This patient group will undoubtedly contain patients that will ultimately relapse, but how do we identify these patients and differentiate them from those that have been cured?

Recent data suggest that markers such as bcl2 and bcl6 may be the key in helping to identify those patients that will eventually recur. No consensus exists as to what follow up should take place in the PET negative normal posttherapy scan. It is clear that some of the low-grade indolent non-Hodgkin's lymphomas can be kept on a "watch and wait" program with little to be lost in withholding therapy until the tumor declares itself clinically. Other low grade lesions will undergo transformation to a more aggressive lymphoma, and these patients benefit from early intervention. The first sign of a transformation can be the increase in the glucose uptake as measured by the SUV. More research is required to clearly identify the role that PET/CT surveillance may have and to confirm any link between tumor markers, FDG uptake and recurrent disease.

AREAS OF POSSIBLE CONFUSION

There have been reports of false-negative PET/CT scanning in relation to certain lymphoma subtypes, such as MALT lymphomas and small lymphocytic NHL. Further inaccurate assessment can be made in relation to the timing of the posttherapy scan. Scanning to soon may result in a false-negative scan, as the tumor is not eradicated but only temporarily stunned. Scanning to late may result in macrophage activity being interpreted as disease—a false-positive scan.

Other possible areas of confusion are post therapy thymic uptake and diffuse bone marrow uptake in those patients receiving granulocyte stimulating factor. Often physiologic metabolic activity in the thymus reflects rebound hyperplasia after chemotherapy or radiotherapy. This effect is more commonly seen in children and young adults. Granulocyte simulating factor can cause such profound metabolic activity within the skeletal system that a coexixting tumor may be difficult to identify. Variable cardiac and bowel activity can be seen in individuals from scan to scan.

Lymphoma involving the central nervous system can be difficult to diagnose due to the intense physiologic uptake of FDG within the brain and cortical gray matter in particular. The future promise of other PET products, such as carbon-11 show promise for accurate imaging of the CNS.

Watch Out for

False-positive causes	False-negative causes
Infection	MALT lymphoma
Inflammation	Lymphocytic NHL
Cardiac/bowel uptake	GSF
Thymic hyperplasia stunning	Posttherapy tumor

FIGURE 3.19. Extensive brown fat activiation.

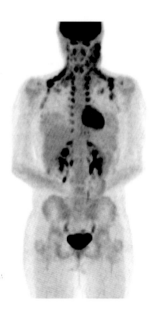

Figure 3.19 is the MIP image of a patient with extensive brown fat activation in the neck, axilla, mediastinum, and upper abdomen. Figure 3.20 is an axial view showing the symmetric uptake in the fat (black areas outside the lungs) within the neck and axilla.

> **Top Tip**
> Brown fat activation can cause confusion and care must be taken to ensure that each area of uptake corresponds to fat. Activated brown fat is seen more commonly in thin individuals during the winter months, but there is also an increased incidence in women and in patients suffering from lymphoma.

Figures 3.21 to 3.23 are AP and lateral MIP views of a patient who was taking granulocyte stimulating factor at the time of the PET/CT. The marrow is so active that little FDG is taken up into any structure other than active bone marrow. There have been reports of tumors being missed due to this effect. There-fore, if possible, a PET/CT should not be performed while the

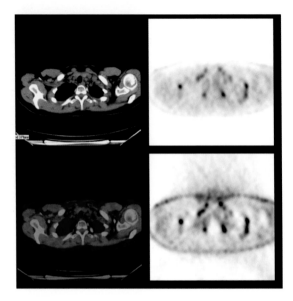

FIGURE 3.20. Extensive brown fat in the neck and axilla bilaterally.

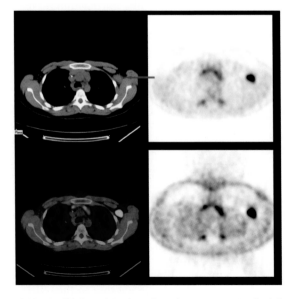

FIGURE 3.21. An FDG positive lymph node is present in the left axilla.

FIGURE 3.22. Intense marrow activation following granulocyte stimulating factor.

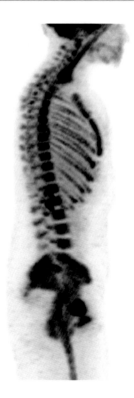

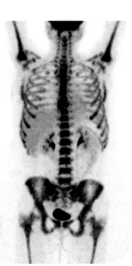

FIGURE 3.23. Another example of intense marrow activation following granulocyte stimulating factor.

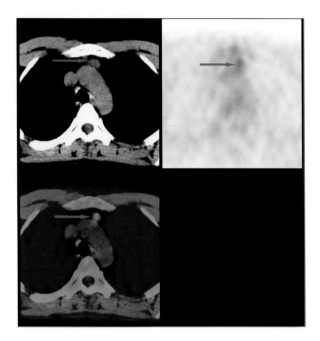

FIGURE 3.24. Incidental thymic rebound hyperplasia following chemotherapy. The arrow points to the thymus, with FDG uptake seen on the PET study.

patient is taking marrow stimulants. Figure 3.24 is an image of the thymus showing low-grade FDG uptake following chemotherapy. This is a common phenomenon related to rebound hyperplasia after initial stunning of the thyroid gland. This is most commonly seen in children and young adults, as beyond this age the thymus tends to involute.

MANAGEMENT CHANGE AS A RESULT OF PET/CT

Many published studies over the last few years indicate significant stage and management changes as a result of PET scanning. Schoder et al showed changes of stage and management of over 40% but other studies reveal changes in the range 10 to 30%. There is less evidence about the influence of combined PET/CT but one must assume that the impact will be at least as profound as PET alone.

The resultant effect has been for more aggressive therapies to be given in those patients with recurrent or residual disease.

In addition, there will also be a decrease in inappropriate chemotherapy to those patients who have a fibrotic residual mass rather than active disease. The long-term impact will also be a reduction in the secondary malignancies induced by chemotherapy regimes.

PET/CT has proved invaluable as an imaging tool for the staging, restaging, and response to therapy. The role of PET/CT in disease surveillance and in radiotherapy planning has yet to be clearly defined. The future role of non-FDG PET/CT shows promise particularly in the staging and management of CNS lymphoma.

Chapter 4
Esophageal and Gastric Cancer

INTRODUCTION

Esophageal cancer is the ninth most common malignancy in the world, and its incidence is rising rapidly particularly in developing countries. Many etiological factors have been shown to be associated with this type of cancer.

Smoking and excess alcohol intake are felt to contribute directly to many cases, but there is a wide geographic, socioeconomic, and racial prevalence of this disease. Two main histological subtypes exist: squamous cell cancer, which primarily affects the upper two-thirds of the esophagus, and adenocarcinoma, which normally is found in the lower third. Less than 40 years ago, only 10% of esophageal cancer was the adenocarcinoma variety but in some areas it makes up over 50% of all new cases. The reasons for this are not fully understood, but are felt to relate to predisposing factors such as Barrett's esophagus, gastroesophageal reflux, and possibly previous mediastinal radiotherapy. The incidence of squamous cell cancer is also on the rise and is strongly related to alcohol and tobacco consumption.

Squamous cell carcinoma	Adenocarcinoma
70% of all cases	25% of all cases
Upper 2/3 esophagus	Lower 1/3 esophagus
Linked to alcohol and tobacco	Linked to Barrett's
Less than 50% of NEW cases	More than 50% of NEW cases

The staging of esophageal cancer is by the TNM staging scheme outlined in Table 4.1. Although there is up to 50% 5-year survival with limited stage disease, unfortunately very few patients present this early. More than 80% of patients present with stage III or IV disease (most are stage IV), with an appalling 5-year survival of less than 5%. The overall 5-year survival is only 10%.

TABLE 4.1. TNM Classification and Staging of Esophageal Cancer

DEFINITION OF TNM

Primary Tumor (T)
TX   Primary tumor cannot be assessed
T0   No evidence of primary tumor
Tis Carcinoma *in situ*
T1   Tumor invades lamina propria or submucosa
T2   Tumor invades muscularis propria
T3   Tumor invades adventitia
T4   Tumor invades adjacent structures

Regional Lymph Nodes (N)
NX   Regional lymph nodes cannot be assessed
N0   No regional lymph node metastasis
N1   Regional lymph node metastasis

Distant Metastasis (M)
MX   Distant metastasis cannot be assessed
M0   No distant metastasis
M1   Distant metastasis

Tumors of the lower thoracic esophagus:
M1a   Metastasis in celiac lymph nodes
M1b   Other distant metastasis

Tumors of the midthoracic esophagus:
M1a   Not applicable
M1b   Nonregional lymph nodes and/or other distant metastasis

Tumors of the upper thoracic esophagus:
M1a   Metastasis in cervical nodes
M1b   Other distant metastasis

STAGE GROUPING			
Stage 0	Tis	N0	M0
Stage I	T1	N0	M0
Stage IIA	T2	N0	M0
	T3	N0	M0
Stage IIB	T1	N1	M0
	T2	N1	M0
Stage III	T3	N1	M0
	T4	Any N	M0
Stage IV	Any T	Any N	M1
Stage IVA	Any T	Any N	M1a
Stage IVB	Any T	Any N	M1b

Source: Used with the permission of the American Joint Committee on Cancer (AJCC), Chicago, Illinois. The original source for this material is the AJCC Cancer Staging Manual, Sixth Edition (2002) published by Springer-New York, www.springeronline.com.

Accurate staging is essential, as surgery is reserved for stages I, IIA, IIB, and occasionally stage III. Surgery increases the overall 5-year survival, but the perisurgical mortality rate is as high as 10%. Chemotherapy, radiotherapy, or combined chemoradiotherapy may be offered as an alternative to surgery in certain cases. The exact role for adjuvant and neoadjuvant chemotherapy is still to be decided. Stage IV disease is considered inoperable and palliative therapy is given (chemotherapy, radiotherapy, tumor stenting).

Top Tip

Stage I, Stage II	Treat surgically	Up to 50% 5-year survival
Stage III	? Surgical? Chemotherapy/ Radiotherapy	
Stage IV	Palliative treatment	Very poor prognosis

The gold standard for assessment of the primary tumor (T stage) is endoscopic ultrasound (EUS). This modality is the most accurate at assessing the depth of invasion into the esophageal wall and identifying local nodes. EUS can stage the primary tumor with an accuracy of between 75 and 95%, but it has difficulty in distinguishing T2 and T3 invasion in some cases.

Although ultrasound is excellent at demonstrating local nodes, it is less accurate at identifying which of these nodes actually are malignant. It can do this with an accuracy of approximately 55%. In addition, the penetration of the ultrasound wave allows good visualization of the left lobe of liver and any nodes around the celiac axis. Beyond this the penetration is insufficient to allow accurate staging.

Contrast enhanced CT scanning has been used to help stage patients with esophageal cancer. CT is useful for the detection of liver or distant metastatic disease, but it is comparatively poor in the staging of the primary tumor and local lymph nodes. At surgery, a significant number of patients are found to have more advanced disease than had been indicated by presurgical imaging and examination. Surgical treatment of esophageal cancer has a high associated mortality rate (up to

20%), and it essential to avoid unnecessary surgery if at all possible.

The primary role for PET/CT in esophageal cancer is in the detection of distant metastases and demonstration of recurrent disease. PET/CT has been shown to be the most sensitive and specific modality in the detection of distant disease with many studies reporting sensitivities of more than 90% in comparison to only 40 to 70% with CT.

Case 1
This is a patient with a known diagnosis of distal esophageal adenocarcinoma.

Figure 4.1 is an MIP image of a patient in whom no distant metastatic disease was identified using routine staging. A small coeliac axis node was seen on CT but was felt to be normal because of size criteria. The MIP identifies abnormal esophageal uptake in keeping with the known tumor (red arrow) but also reveals abnormal uptake in the ribs (black arrows), and a mediastinal node and a celiac axis node (yellow arrows). In Figure 4.2, the abnormal FDG uptake is confined to the esophagus and no distant metabolically active disease is demonstrated.

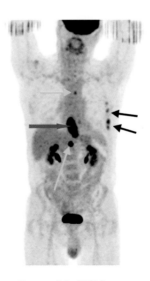

FIGURE 4.1. MIP image.

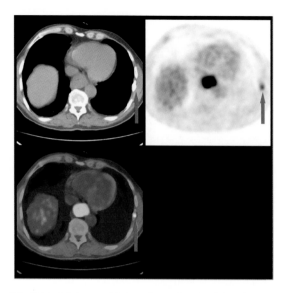

FIGURE 4.1. (A) Axial Image. The uptake within the left-sided ribs (arrow) represent incidental uptake in traumatic rib fractures resulting from a recent fall.

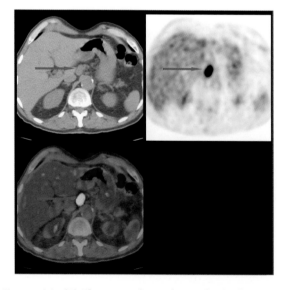

FIGURE 4.1. (B) The arrow shows the involved celiac node.

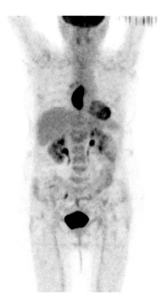

FIGURE 4.2. Abnormal esophageal uptake without distant FDG positive macroscopic disease.

PET has a relatively poor sensitivity for the detection of involved locoregional nodes and can not compete with endoscopic ultrasound in this arena. PET does, however, show a very high specificity in the detection of local nodal involvement with studies indicating specificities of more than 90%. PET/CT has reduced unnecessary surgical procedures by the noninvasive detection of distant metastases. These patients are then treated with palliative chemotherapy or chemoradiotherapy and spared gruelling surgery.

PRIMARY TUMOR (T) STAGING
- **Endoscopic ultrasound:** The gold standard for T staging, with an accuracy of >85%.
- **CT:** Not a reliable indicator of primary tumor resectability.
- **PET/CT:** Most tumors have a high uptake of FDG, but small T1 lesions and gastroesophageal tumors can be missed. Accurate T staging is not possible.

NODAL (N) STAGING
- **Endoscopic ultrasound:** Better than CT for staging local nodes, with an overall accuracy of approximately 85% for

assessment of T staging and 55% for local N staging. Not accurate for distant nodal or metastatic spread because of limited penetration of the ultrasound wave.

- **CT:** Relatively poor accuracy for local nodal involvement (approximately 40%).
- **PET/C:** Higher sensitivity than CT and very high specificity (>90%)

METASTATIC (M) STAGING
- **Endoscopic ultrasound:** Not routinely used for this indication but can assess the left lobe of liver and the celiac axis.
- **CT:** Overall accuracy of 40 to 60% for staging and is best used for hepatic and adrenal metastases.
- **PET/CT:** Superior to both CT and EUS combined in the diagnosis of stage 4 disease with an accuracy of over 85%.

Case 2
Figure 4.3 illustrates the case of a patient with mid and lower esophageal tumor. The PET/CT scan clearly reveals that the disease has spread to involve nodal groups both above and below the diaphragm as well as the liver.

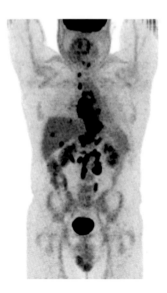

FIGURE 4.3. Tumor extending from mid to distal esophagus. It has spread to nodes above and below the diaphragm, as well as to the liver.

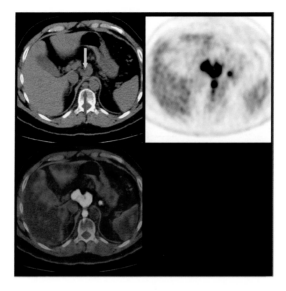

FIGURE 4.3. (A) Active celiac axis (yellow) and rectrocrural nodes (red).

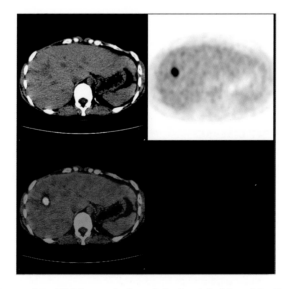

FIGURE 4.3. (B) Metastatic deposit in the right lobe of the liver.

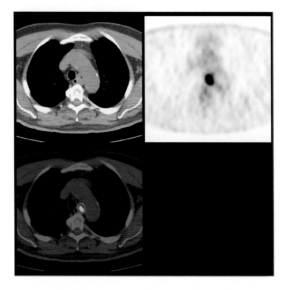

FIGURE 4.3. (C) Metastatic deposit in the mediastinum.

Top Tip
Lower esophageal tumors tend to have nodal spread to below the diaphragm and involve the coeliac and superior mesenteric nodes and the liver. Tumors of the upper third of the esophagus tend to involve the mediastinal nodes and can spread superiorly into the neck via the internal jugular chain.

RECURRENT DISEASE

PET/CT has been shown to be the most effective tool in the diagnosis of recurrent disease particularly around the anastomotic site. Figure 4.4 is a coronal fused image and a single axial image through the mediastinum in a patient who had a previous esophagectomy following diagnosis of an adenocarcinoma of the distal esophagus. The image reveals an area of abnormal FDG uptake in the neo-esophagus. This region extends along the neoesophagus as seen on the coronal view and the arrow points to the FDG uptake on the axial image. This was shown to contain malignant cells on biopsy. Incidental note is made of the right sided pleural effusion.

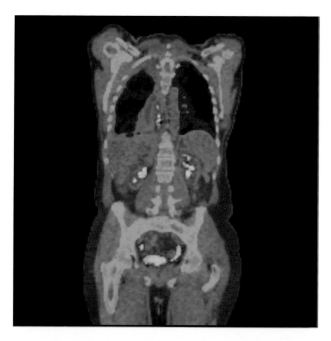

FIGURE 4.4. Coronal fused view of a recurrence in the neoesophagus.

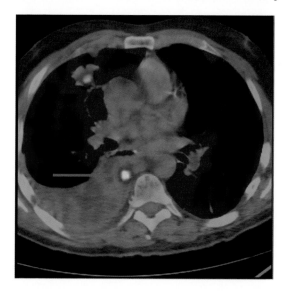

FIGURE 4.4. (a) Axial view demonstrating recurrent disease around the anastomotic site (arrow).

RESPONSE TO THERAPY

Recent literature indicates the metabolic changes that take place following chemotherapy, as reflected in the appearances of the PET/CT scan. Many centers now offer neoadjuvant chemotherapy to those patients considered operable following staging with PET/CT (as well as CT and EUS). PET/CT scans repeated after the chemotherapy but prior to surgery appear to correlate with histology following resection. In other words, those tumors that appear to have a PET response to chemotherapy, as indicated by a reduction in SUV, also appear to have a histological response. These findings appear to hold only for esophageal tumors but not for junctional or gastric lesions (see later in this chapter).

Case 3

Figure 4.5 and Figure 4.6 are the pretherapy and post-therapy MIP images in a patient who received neoadjuvant chemotherapy. The maximum FDG uptake reduced from an SUV of 15 prior to chemotherapy to an SUV of 2 posttherapy. The patient had an esophagectomy and remains well 24 months after surgery.

> **Top Tip**
> Junctional tumors may have very low-grade uptake and resemble only physiological patterns.

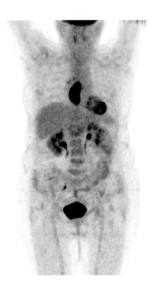

FIGURE 4.5. Intense FDG uptake in esophageal tumor with SUV 15.

FIGURE 4.6. Post-neoadjuvant therapy
SUV reduced from 15 to 2.

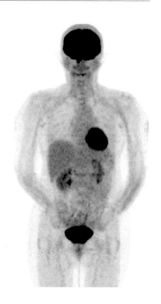

GASTRO-ESOPHAGEAL JUNCTIONAL TUMORS
The use of PET/CT in the detection of junctional tumors has been questioned by some practitioners. It is clear that some gastro-esophageal tumors have only very low-grade associated FDG uptake and prove difficult to detect on either PET or CT. Figure 4.7 demonstrates the relatively low-grade uptake seen in a known gastro-esophageal junctional tumor. The degree of uptake within tumors at this site can be very low. In fact the appearances can be similar to physiological low grade distal esophageal uptake sometimes found.

GASTRIC TUMORS
Because of the normal physiological uptake to FDG into the gastric wall and the subsequent excretion into the lumen of the digestive tract, it can be difficult to detect small gastric tumors. There is emerging evidence that suggests that PET/CT would best be deployed for the detection of distant metastatic spread from gastric tumors. The most common tumor found in the stomach is adenocarcinoma. The risk factors for this include, diet, ade-nomatous polyps, and pernicious anemia.

Gastric lymphoma is the second most common malignancy of the stomach and often begins following an accumulation of mucosa associated lymphoid tissue in response to H. pylori infection, the so-called MALT lymphoma. The incidence of AIDS related gastric lymphoma is increasing worldwide.

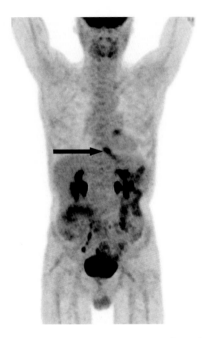

FIGURE 4.7. Relatively low uptake in a gastroeophageal juntional tumor (arrow).

The role of PET/CT is better defined in the diagnosis and management of gastric lymphoma and its use is established in staging, restaging, response to therapy and prognosis (see Chapter 3).

Figures 4.8 and 4.9 are two examples that indicate the range of intensity found within gastric adenocarcinoma. Figure 4.8 is an axial image through the level of the stomach and it reveals a small focus of uptake on the proximal aspect of the greater curvature of the stomach. This was the site of an adenocarcinoma but the uptake is no grater than physiological uptake found in some patients. Figure 4.9 is an axial view through another patient with intense uptake in the stomach corresponding to the tumor. Notice the slight thickening of the wall at this site. Figure 4.10 is the corresponding MIP image of the patient seen in Figure 4.9.

Case 4
A patient with a known gastric tumor considered resectable following staging with CT, EUS, and laparoscopy.

Figure 4.11 shows that the PET/CT scan revealed only low-grade uptake at the site of the gastric primary but extensive small

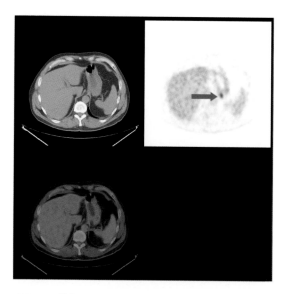

FIGURE 4.8. Small focus of uptake within a gastric adenocarcinoma.

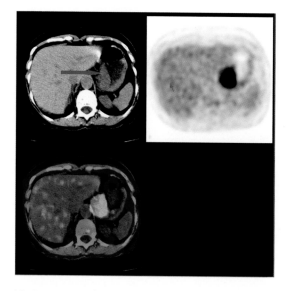

FIGURE 4.9. Intense uptake within a gastric adenocarcinoma. Note the associated stomach wall thickening (arrow).

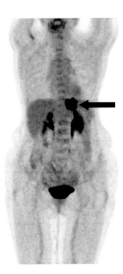

FIGURE 4.10. The MIP image of the patient in Figure 4.9. Note the intense FDG uptake in the left upper quadrant corresponding to the gastric tumor (arrow).

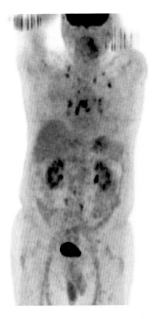

FIGURE 4.11. MIP image revealing extensive neck and mediastinal nodal involvement.

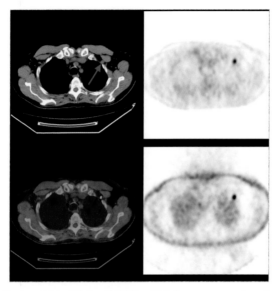

FIGURE 4.11. (A) Small FDG avid left retropectoral node.

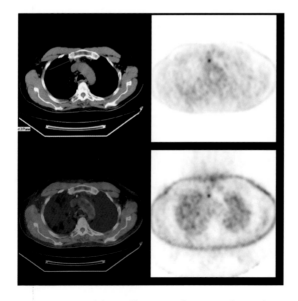

FIGURE 4.11. (B) Small FDG avid prevascular node.

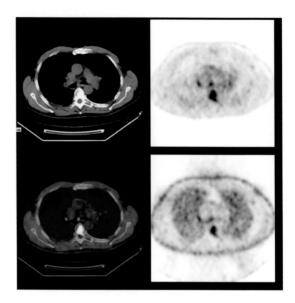

FIGURE 4.11. (C) **FDG** avid vertebral body metastatic deposit.

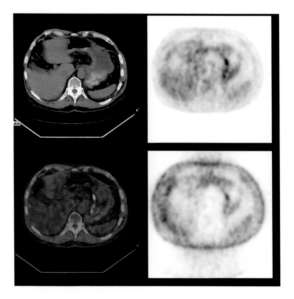

FIGURE 4.11. (D) **FDG** uptake within the gastric primary is relatively low grade. This degree of intensity can be mimicked by normal physiological gastric uptake.

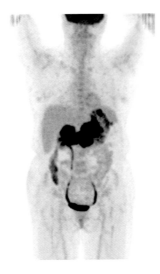

FIGURE 4.12. Intense uptake seen in a gastric lymphoma before therapy.

volume disease within the mediastinum and neck which went undetected with conventional imaging. Figure 4.11 demonstrates small volume nodal disease, which was not detected using conventional staging. Figure 4.11D specifically demonstrates the gastric primary which has relatively low-grade FDG uptake.

> **Top Tip**
> These cases illustrate well the variable degree of uptake found within gastric adenocarcinoma and the difficulties with accurate staging. What has also been demonstrated is the possible use of PET/CT in the detection of metastatic spread from a gastric primary.

Figure 4.12 and Figure 4.13 are the MIP and axial views in a patient with a MALT lymphoma of the stomach. These patients are not treated with surgery as the tumor tends to respond well to chemotherapy. Figure 4.14 is the posttherapy MIP scan and it reveals a complete metabolic response to treatment.

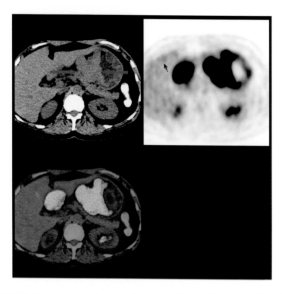

FIGURE 4.13. Intense uptake seen in a gastric lymphoma before therapy. Note the significant expophytic wall thickening often seen in gastrointestinal lymphoma (arrow).

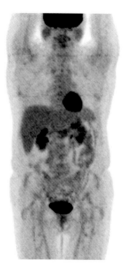

FIGURE 4.14. Normal uptake in the same patient after therapy. Note the complete metabolic response to therapy.

Top Tip
<u>Indications for PET/CT</u>
Preoperative staging to identify nodal and disseminated metastases
Demonstration of recurrent disease
Assess the response to therapy including neoadjuvant chemotherapy

And possibly . . .
Predicting response to therapy and overall prognosis
but . . .
be careful in the use of PET/CT in gastric malignancy other than lymphoma

<u>False Positive and False Negative- Potential Pitfalls</u>

False negative
Small T1 lesions
Local nodes applied close to the primary
Linitis plastica
Peritoneal mets
False positive
Gastritis
Barrett's
Esophagitis
Normal contracted stomach
Physiological uptake gastric outlet

Figure 4.15 is an axial image showing low-grade uptake of FDG within the pyloric outlet. This can be found as a normal physiological finding because of the excretion of FDG into the bowel lumen. In this case, however, the uptake was associated with an area of pyloric and proximal duodenal gastritis.

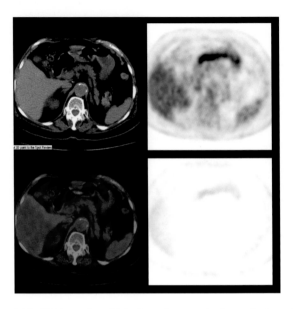

FIGURE 4.15. FDG uptake within the pylorus realted to pyloric and duodenal gastritis. A similar physiological finding is sometimes seen because of excretion of FDG into the bowel lumen.

MANAGEMENT CHANGE

Centers with access to PET/CT for the preoperative staging of esophageal cancer have shown profound changes in patient management as a result of the PET/CT findings. Some have had a reduction in esophagectomy rate of more than 40%. Recent work has suggested that PET/CT carried out pre- and postneoadjuvant chemotherapy can predict those patients that have histologically responded to the therapeutic regime.

Chapter 5
Colorectal Cancer

INTRODUCTION

Colorectal cancer (CRC) is the second most common cause of death from cancer in both the UK and the US. The incidence increases with age, and the disease is much more common in Western industrialized countries that have a high-fat, low-fiber diet. In most cases, CRC develops over a period of years in a preexisting adenomatous polyp (the "adenoma-carcinoma sequence"). Knowledge of this pathway has led to the development of screening programs using colonoscopy or barium enema. The size of the polyp determines the risk of malignant change; only a small percentage of polyps will develop into cancers. Those less than 1 cm have less than a 1% chance of containing malignant cells, whereas half of those over 2 cm are malignant. Approximately 3% of patients with colorectal cancer will have a second or synchronous tumor at the time of presentation.

Top Tip
Incidence: 30 per 100,000
Peak Age: 60–69 years
Male = Female
Histology: 95% Adenocarcinoma
5-year survival 50%
Site: 40% rectal, 60% colonic

RISK FACTORS AND PROGNOSIS

The risk factors for CRC are:

1. Age
2. Diet
3. Polyps
4. Chronic Ulcerative Colitis
5. Familial polyposis coli (FAP)

TABLE 5.1 TNM Classification and Stage Gouping

DEFINITION OF TNM

The same classification is used for both clinical and pathologic staging.

Primary Tumor (T)
TX   Primary tumor cannot be assessed
T0   No evidence of primary tumor
Tis Carcinoma *in situ*: intraepithelial or invasion of lamina propria*
T1   Tumor invades submusosa
T2   Tumor invades muscularis propria
T3   Tumor invades through the muscularis propria into the subserosa, or into non-peritonealized pericolic or perirectal tissues
T4   Tumor directly invades other organs or structures, and/or perforates visceral peritoneum**,***

*Note: Tis includes cancer cells confined within the glandular basement membrane (intraepithelial) or lamina propria (intramucosal) with no extension through the muscularis mucosae into the submucosa.
**Note: Direct invasion in T4 includes invasion of other segments of the colorectum by way of the serosa; for example, invasion of the sigmoid colon by a carcinoma of the cecum.
***Tumor that is adherent to other organs or structures, macroscophically, is classified T4. However, if no tumor is present in the adhesion, microscopically, the classification should be pT3. The V and L substaging should be used to identify the presence or absence of vascular or lymphatic invasion.

Regional Lymph Nodes (N)
NX   Regional lymph nodes cannot be assessed
N0   No regional lymph node metastasis
N1   Metastasis in 1 to 3 regional lymph nodes
N2   Metastasis in 4 or more regional lymph nodes

Note: A tumor nodule in the pericolorectal adipose tissue of a primary carcinoma without histologic evidence of residual lymph node in the nodule is classified in the pN category as a regional lymph node metastasis if the nodule has the form and smooth contour of a lymph node. If the nodule has an irregular contour, it should be classified in the T category and also coded as V1 (microscopic venous invasion) or as V2 (if it was grossly evident), because there is a strong likelihood that it represents venous invasion.

Distant Metastasis (M)
MX   Distant metastasis cannot be assessed
M0   No distant metastasis
M1   Distant metastasis

TABLE 5.1 *Continued*

STAGE GROUPING					
Stage	T	N	M	Dukes*	MAC*
0	Tis	N0	M0	—	—
I	T1	N0	M0	A	A
	T2	N0	M0	A	B1
IIA	T3	N0	M0	B	B2
IIB	T4	N0	M0	B	B3
IIIA	T1–T2	N1	M0	C	C1
IIIB	T3–T4	N1	M0	C	C2/C3
IIIC	Any T	N2	M0	C	C1/C2/C3
IV	Any T	Any N	M1	—	D

*Dukes B is a composite of better (T3 N0 M0) and worse (T4 N0 M0) prognostic groups, as is Dukes C (Any TN1 M0 and Any T N2 M0). MAC is the modified Astler-Coller classification.
Note: The y prefix is to be used for those cancers that are classified after pretreatment, whereas the r prefix is to be used for those cancers that have recurred.
Source: Used with the permission of the American Joint Committee on Cancer (AJCC), Chicago, Illinois. The original source for this material is the AJCC Cancer Staging Manual, Sixth Edition (2002) published by Springer-New York, www.springeronline.com.

6. Hereditary nonpolyposis colorectal cancer (HNPCC)
7. Previous history of bowel cancer (metachronous tumor)

The prognosis depends on the stage of the disease. Accurate staging is important to determine the best treatment for each individual patient. The TNM and Dukes staging schemes are outlined in Tables 5.1 and 5.2.

Even in cases with known metastases, the treatment is usually surgical. This will relieve local symptoms and help prevent possible obstruction. The spread of disease is slightly different in colonic and rectal cancers. Colonic spread is generally through the

TABLE 5.2. Dukes Staging

Stage	Description	5-Year Survival
A	Confined to bowel wall	80%
B	Penetration of wall but no lymph node involvement	50%
C1	Lymph nodes involved but not beyond the highest point of vascular ligation	40%
C2	Lymph nodes involved beyond the highest point of vascular ligation	12%
D	Distant metastases	<5%

bowel wall and along the lymphatic chain towards the liver and lungs. Low rectal tumors tend to spread laterally and involve the local nodes. As a result, some rectal lesions will benefit from pre-operative radiotherapy. Radiotherapy can also be useful in some inoperable or recurrent cancers. Chemotherapy has so far proved rather ineffectual with objective transient responses seen in a minority of patients, but there is some evidence that post surgical adjuvant therapy may be valuable. There is a higher rate of local recurrence with rectal cancer compared with colonic cancer, and recent evidence would recommend a combined postoperative regime of chemotherapy and radiotherapy for these patients.

Liver metastases can be successfully removed surgically in some cases or treated with radiofrequency ablation in others. Some hepatic metastases may respond to an infusion of chemotherapy via the hepatic veins. Overall, there has been a slight decrease in the mortality rate over the past few years. This may possibly reflect the impact of screening, improvement in diet or indeed the introduction of combined therapies for treatment and management.

> **Top Tip**
> The disease may be cured by surgery with approximately 50% 5-year survival rate. Radiotherapy reduces the risk of local recurrence in rectal cancer.
> Liver metastases can be cured by surgery, radiofrequency ablation and possibly hepatic vein infusion of chemotherapy.
> Chemotherapy and radiotherapy are used for palliation.

COMMON SITES OF METASTASES

The most common sites of metastases are the:

1. Liver
2. Lung
3. Retroperitoneum
4. Ovaries
5. Peritoneum

THE ROLE OF IMAGING IN COLORECTAL CANCER

Secondary prevention of disease in high-risk groups has had some success with the use of sigmoidoscopy and tests for fecal occult blood. Measurement of the tumor marker carcinoembryonic antigen (CEA) has proved insensitive for the detection of early cancer but may be more sensitive in recurrent disease.

Noninvasive tests, such as CT, ultrasound, and MRI do not play a major role in the diagnosis and certainly not in the screening of colorectal cancer. They are more commonly used to stage the disease prior to surgery and restage it after subsequent intervention.

The use of PET/CT is not generally advocated for the initial diagnosis and staging of colorectal cancer. Despite the fact that PET alone has a very high sensitivity in the detection of primary tumors (>95%), its specificity is relatively low because of false-positive uptake of FDG in areas of postsurgical inflammation, such as an inflammatory bowel, and the fact that some individuals can have focal, segmental, or diffuse areas of physiological FDG excretion into the bowel lumen that can cause confusion. In addition, both CT and PET may miss the involvement of local nodes which are occasionally found only when both PET and CT are viewed simultaneously.

As we have seen in esophageal cancer, neither PET nor CT can provide an accurate T-stage assessment of wall invasion. PET/CT has been shown to be the most accurate modality for the detection of distant metastases but the lack of scanners prevents most patients from being scanned before initial surgery.

The major role for PET/CT has been in the restaging of recurrent disease and the detection of metastases. The most common site of recurrent disease is within the liver, followed closely by lung and anastomotic local recurrence. Of the patients who are believed to be surgically cured, one-third will have a recurrence within 2 years and 25% of recurrences are isolated to a single site and are potentially curable.

PET/CT has been shown to detect hepatic recurrence with a greater overall accuracy than CT, MRI or CT portography. Because the resection of liver metastasis has been shown to improve overall patient mortality by up to 25%, it is essential that all lesions are demonstrated during preoperative imaging. In the detection of distant metastatic disease PET/CT finds approximately 30% more disease than CT alone.

Top Tip
Accuracy in detection of CRC recurrence

	Sensitivity	Specificity
PET	94	87
CT	79	73

MANAGEMENT CHANGE

PET is significantly more accurate than CT in detecting recurrent CRC and changes management in approximately one third of cases.

It is well recognized that conventional imaging fails to detect a significant number of metastatic deposits in the liver and fares even worse with extrahepatic deposits. Studies have shown that PET/CT has a greater sensitivity and specificity for the detection of hepatic metastases than any other modality, and its diagnostic accuracy greatly exceeds CT in the detection of extra hepatic disease.

PET/CT can be deployed in the detection of tumor recurrence in patients with an unexplained rise in CEA and negative imaging findings with other modalities. Several studies have been published assessing the use of PET and PET/CT in monitoring the response of various therapeutic regimes.

PET/CT is also useful in distinguishing postoperative fibrotic change from recurrent or residual disease. Again, the timing of the scan is essential, as early scanning may lead to false-positive results because of FDG uptake within active macrophage activity within postoperative inflammatory change. Waiting until 6 months have elapsed from surgery is recommended before embarking on a PET/CT scan to assess local recurrence.

PET is a sensitive method for monitoring the effects of radiotherapy, but its specificity is somewhat limited by early radiation induced inflammatory responses. This problem can be overcome by waiting until this effect subsides. Imaging 3 to 6 months after radiotherapy usually avoids any inflammatory response.

Early PET responses to chemotherapy (e.g., as soon as after 4 weeks of treatment), have been shown to discriminate between responders and nonresponders. The reduction in SUV posttherapy gives a guide to the degree of tumor responsiveness and overall prognosis. Similar data has been presented about PET assessment of the response of hepatic chemoembolisation, successful treatment being marked by a significant reduction in FDG uptake.

> **Top Tip**
> Clinical Indications for PET in CRC
> 1. Assessment of recurrent disease
> 2. Prior to metastectomy for colorectal cancer
> 3. Assessment of tumor response to chemo/radiotherapy
> 4. Assessment of a mass that is difficult to biopsy
> 5. Unexplained rising CEA in patients with a history of colorectal cancer and normal conventional imaging.

False-Positives
1. Physiological uptake
2. Inflammation (e.g., diverticulitis, colitis)
3. Polyps
4. Stoma site/postoperative changes

False-Negatives
1. small volume disease
2. mucinous secreting tumors
3. Peritoneal metastases
4. Carcinoid tumors

Case 1

One of the most important indications for PET-CT in colorectal cancer is in the assessment of recurrent disease. This patient had previously undergone a resection of a midsigmoid carcinoma. A follow-up CT scan demonstrated a soft tissue mass adjacent to the anastomosis, CT or MRI do not make it possible to differentiate postoperative fibrosis from recurrent disease. There is however high-grade uptake of FDG within this lesion and a metabolically active right lower lobe pulmonary nodule both of which indicate the presence of recurrent disease.

Figure 5.1 is an MIP image showing abnormal FDG uptake superior to the bladder (arrow) and an active focus in the right lung base (arrow). Note the partially extravasated FDG in the right arm. Figure 5.2 shows the sagittal (left) and axial (right) views of the FDG positive presacral mass (arrows), which is seen in the MIP image in Figure 5.1. Figure 5.3 shows coronal and axial views of the right lower lobe nodule with FDG uptake and representing an active pulmonary metastatic deposit.

Case 2

This patient had previously undergone a right hemicolectomy for a carcinoma of the cecum. A follow-up CT scan demonstrated two metastases in the the right lobe of the liver, but there was no other evidence of recurrent disease. Resection of isolated liver metastases is potentially curative in this situation, but a PET/CT scan demonstrated evidence of multiple bilobar liver metastases that had not been detected on CT. The patient therefore received palliative therapy and did not undergo a hepatic resection. Figures 5.4 to 5.8 are the MIP and selected axial and coronal views demonstrating some of the 12 (at least) lesions identified within the liver.

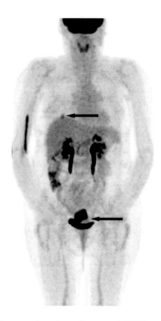

FIGURE 5.1. MIP image showing abnormal FDG uptake superior to the bladder (arrow) and an active focus in the right lung base (arrow). Note the partially extravasated FDG in the right arm.

Case 3

This patient had a history of colorectal cancer. Postoperative follow-up showed that the CEA was rising, but no evidence of recurrence was found on CT. The subsequent PET scan however, shows a single abnormal focus of FDG uptake in the liver which was treated with a metastectomy. Figures 5.9 and 5.10 are MIP and single axial views demonstrating a solitary metastatic deposit within the right lobe of liver.

Case 4

This patient has a known adenocarcinoma of the rectum, but had a PET/CT scan that revealed intense abnormal uptake in the cecum. This lesion was a synchronous primary tumor of the caecum. The incidence of such synchronous lesions is about 3%. Figures 5.11 and 5.12 are the AP and lateral MIP views showing the cecal and rectal lesions respectively. The corresponding axial views are seen in Figures 5.13 and 5.14.

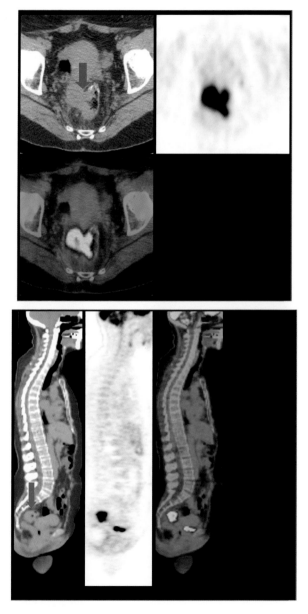

FIGURE 5.2. Sagittal (top) and axial (bottom) views of the FDG positive presacral mass.

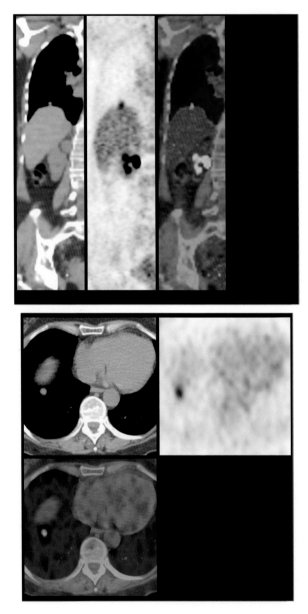

FIGURE 5.3. Coronal and axial views of the right lower lobe nodule showing FDG uptake.

FIGURE 5.4. MIP image revealing bilobar liver metastases.

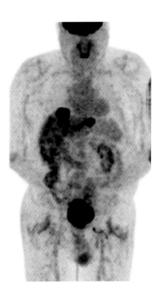

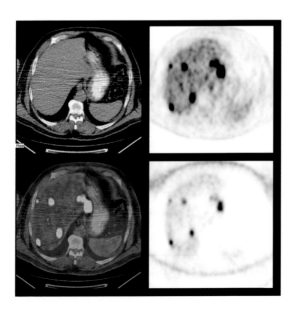

FIGURE 5.5. At least five metabolically active lesions are demonstrated on this single axial view.

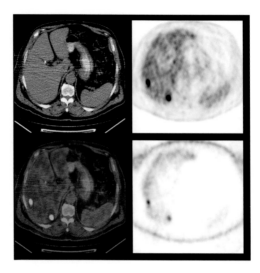

FIGURE 5.6. Two further right lobe metastases.

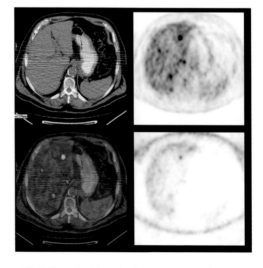

FIGURE 5.7. Left and right lobe lesions seen in the axial section.

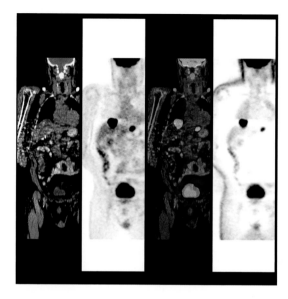

FIGURE 5.8. Left and right lobe lesions seen in the coronal section.

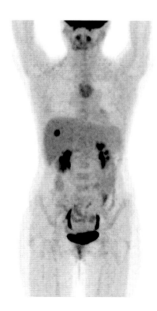

FIGURE 5.9. Rising CEA with normal CT findings. A FDG positive deposit is seen in the liver.

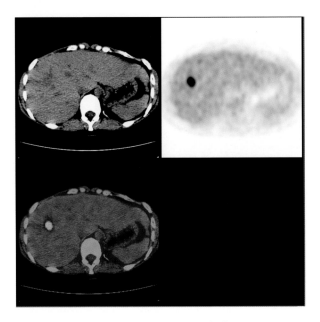

FIGURE 5.10. Rising CEA with normal CT findings. A FDG positive deposit is seen in the right lobe of the liver.

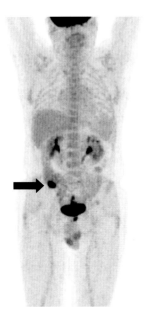

FIGURE 5.11. AP MIP view shows the abnormal uptake in the cecal pole (arrow).

FIGURE 5.12. Lateral MIP view showing abnormal uptake lying behind the bladder (arrow).

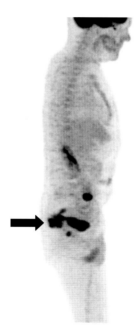

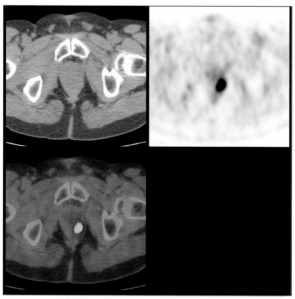

FIGURE 5.13. Rectal primary lesion.

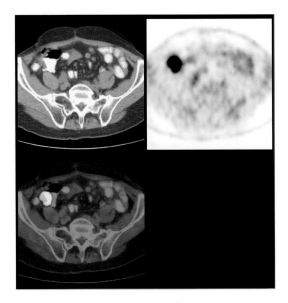

FIGURE 5.14. Synchronous primary within the cecum.

Case 5

In this case, there had been a recent rise in the CEA, but no CT abnormality had been detected. The patient had a previous resection for colonic carcinoma. The PET/CT MIP scan reveals four abnormal foci of FDG uptake, as seen in Figure 5.15 (the lesions are marked with arrows). Figures 5.16 and 5.17 show that the uptake resides in small soft tissue nodules in the peritoneum. Lesions like these are poorly detected by CT, as they often lie adjacent to the small bowel or colon, and it is assumed that they represent unenhanced bowel loops.

Case 6

This 54-year-old male presented with a rectal cancer and was staged conventionally with contrast enhanced CT. A subsequent PET/CT scan revealed two active metastatic deposits in the right lobe of the liver and a further unsuspected deposit in the right iliacus muscle. These findings are seen on the MIP image in Figure 5.18. Figure 5.19 is an axial image that clearly shows the metastatic deposit in the right iliacus muscle that was not identified on the staging CT scan.

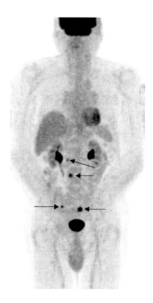

FIGURE 5.15. Rising CEA with normal CT scan. Four abnormal foci of uptake are demonstrated that correspond to peritoneal metastases.

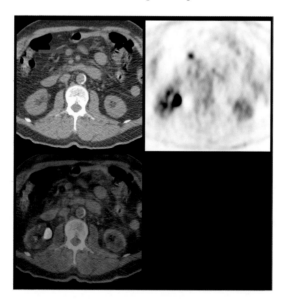

FIGURE 5.16. Rising CEA with normal CT scan. Abnormal focus of uptake within a small soft tissue peritoneal deposit.

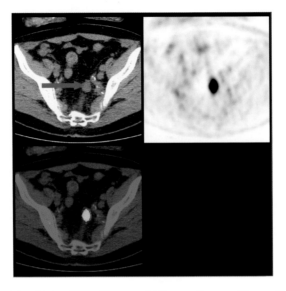

FIGURE 5.17. Rising CEA with normal CT scan. Abnormal focus of uptake within a further pelvic deposit.

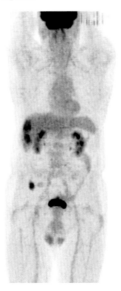

FIGURE 5.18. Rectal cancer with a solitary liver met demonstrated on CT. Two abnormal liver lesions are seen and a soft tissue deposit in the right iliacus muscle.

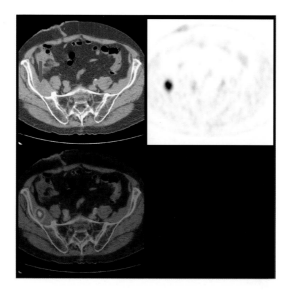

FIGURE 5.19. Rectal cancer with a soltary liver met demonstrated on CT. Metastatic deposit in the right iliacus muscle.

Case 7
The patient had a resection of a sigmoid adenocarcinoma 12 months earlier. Figure 5.20 is the axial image through a presacral mass demonstrated on a postoperative CT scan. The abnormal FDG uptake seen in the presacral mass represented recurrent disease in this case. Postoperative inflammatory change would have been expected to resolve by 6 months.

Case 8
The patient had a resection of a sigmoid adenocarcinoma 12 months earlier. Figures 5.21 to 5.23 show that the CEA, 18 months after surgery, was steadily rising and CT scanning revealed calicified liver and pancreatic tail lesions. The PET/CT scan showed multiple, active, calcified, liver metastases with central photopenic necrosis and both pancreatic tail and paraaortic nodal involvement.

Case 9
Figures 5.24 and 5.25 show the appearances of an inflammatory stricture of the sigmoid colon (red arrow) on lateral MIP view

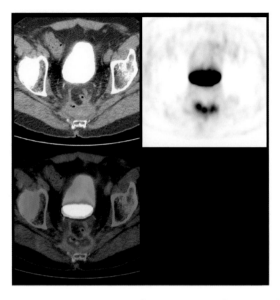

FIGURE 5.20. Postoperative presacral mass. FDG uptake 12 months after surgery indicates recurrence.

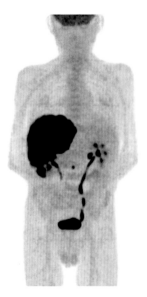

FIGURE 5.21. Previous colonic cancer with calcified liver metastases with central photopenic necrosis and both pancreatic tail and paraaortic involvement.

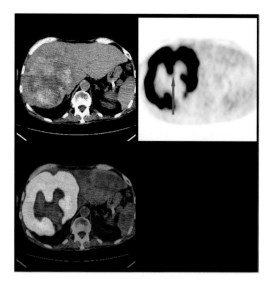

FIGURE 5.22. Previous colonic cancer with calcified liver metastases with central photopenic necrosis and both pancreatic tail and paraaortic involvement.

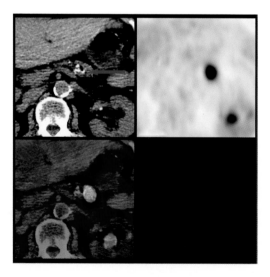

FIGURE 5.23. Previous colonic cancer with calcified liver metastases with central photopenic necrosis and both pancreatic tail and paraaortic involvement.

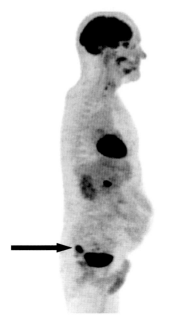

FIGURE 5.24. Lateral MIP view of inflammatory stricture of the sigmoid colon (red arrow).

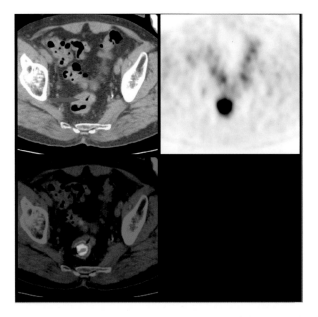

FIGURE 5.25. Axial view of inflammatory stricture of the sigmoid colon (red arrow).

and axial view through the area. Notice the FDG avid wall thickening of the sigmoid colon. This scan shows that inflammatory lesions can also have intense FDG uptake. Remember that, just because a lesion is metabolically active does not mean it is necessarily malignant.

Chapter 6
Head and Neck Cancer

INTRODUCTION

PET/CT is developing an increasing role in the management of head and neck (H&N) epithelial cancers, especially the oropharyngeal, nasopharyngeal, and laryngeal squamous cell cancers that are the most common. Head and neck cancers are the sixth most common malignancy worldwide and make up 2 to 5% of cancers in the population.

Because of their location, they are difficult to treat and usually require a specialized team of surgeons, oncologists, nurses, radiologists, and other allied staff to help in their treatment. Surgery, radiotherapy, and chemoradiotherapy in these patients have profound impact on the patients' feeding, speech, and social well-being. All of this needs to be supported. H&N cancer has an unwarranted poor reputation because of its impact on the day-to-day life of the patient, but the five-year survival of advanced (stage IV) disease is approximately 30%, which is excellent when compared with other epithelial aerodigestive tract malignancies.

Most head and neck cancers are relatively advanced at the time of presentation; less than one-third is Stage I or II. The vast majority (>75%) of these cancers occur in the tongue base or within the tonsillar fossa. Alcohol and tobacco are two etiological factors strongly linked to the promotion of head and neck cancer, and they act in a strongly synergistic way. Patients with heavy tobacco and alcohol consumption often develop a second primary tumur of the lung or esophagus in due course.

The staging, treatment, and prognosis are tumor dependant, but as with most other tumors, early detection and treatment offer the best chance of long-term survival.

There are slight differences in the T-staging descriptors for the various tumor subtypes, but the N and M patterns are the same for all head and neck cancer types. The TNM staging system for oropharyngeal cancer is outlined in Table 6.1. Stage descriptors are shown in Table 6.2.

TABLE 6.1. TNM Classification

DEFINITION OF TNM

Primary Tumor (T)

TX	Primary tumor cannot be assessed
T0	No evidence of primary tumor
Tis	Carcinoma *in situ*
T1	Tumor 2 cm or less in greatest dimension
T2	Tumor more than 2 cm but not more than 4 cm in greatest dimension
T3	Tumor more than 4 cm in greatest dimension
T4 (lip)	Tumor invades through cortical bone, inferior alveolar nerve, floor of mouth, or skin of face, i.e., chin or nose
T4a	(oral cavity) Tumor invades adjacent structures (e.g., through cortical bone, into deep [extrinsic] muscle of tongue [genioglossus, hyoglossus, palatoglossus, and sytloglossus], maxillary sinus, skin of face)
T4b	Tumor invades masticator space, pterygoid plates, or skull base and/or encases internal carotid artery

Note: Superficial erosion alone of bone/tooth socket by gingival primary is not sufficient to classify a tumor as T4.

Regional Lymph Nodes (N)

NX	Regional lymph nodes cannot be assessed
N0	No regional lymph node metastasis
N1	Metastasis in a single ipsilateral lymph node, 3 cm or less in greatest dimension
N2	Metastasis in a single ipsilateral lymph node, more than 3 cm but not more than 6 cm in greatest dimension; or in multiple ipsilateral lymph nodes, none more than 6 cm in greatest dimension; or in bilateral or contralateral lymph nodes, none more than 6 cm in greatest dimension
N2a	Metastasis in single ipsilateral lymph node more than 3 cm but not more than 6 cm in greatest dimension
N2b	Metastasis in multiple ipsilateral lymph nodes, none more than 6 cm in greatest dimension
N2c	Metastasis in bilateral or contralateral lymph nodes, none more than 6 cm in greatest dimension
N3	Metastasis in a lymph node more than 6 cm in greatest dimension

Distant Metastasis (M)

MX	Distant metastasis cannot be assessed
M0	No distant metastasis
M1	Distant metastasis

Source: Used with the permission of the American Joint Committee on Cancer (AJCC), Chicago, Illinois. The original source for this material is the AJCC Cancer Staging Manual, Sixth Edition (2002) published by Springer-New York, www.springeronline.com.

TABLE 6.2. TNM Stage Descriptions

STAGE GROUPING			
Stage 0	Tis	N0	M0
Stage I	T1	N0	M0
Stage II	T2	N0	M0
Stage III	T3	N0	M0
	T1	N1	M0
	T2	N1	M0
	T3	N1	M0
Stage IVA	T4a	N0	M0
	T4a	N1	M0
	T1	N2	M0
	T2	N2	M0
	T3	N2	M0
	T4a	N2	M0
Stage IVB	Any T	N3	M0
	T4b	Any N	M0
Stage IVC	Any T	Any N	M1

Source: Used with the permission of the American Joint Committee on Cancer (AJCC), Chicago, Illinois. The original source for this material is the AJCC Cancer Staging Manual, Sixth Edition (2002) published by Springer-New York, www.springeronline.com.

The pattern of normal FDG uptake in the H&N is complex, and the combination of anatomical and functional information seen in PET/CT has enabled these patterns to be more clearly defined. This has also allowed the quality of the PET/CT to be assessed as never before and has reduced the effects of minor degrees of movement on the quality of the PET images. The anatomy, pathology, and iatrogenic effects of H&N cancer and its treatment are intricate, but the patterns are knowable. We will show you some of these patterns in this chapter.

PET/CT has established itself as important in the detection of local recurrent disease after treatment of head and neck cancer. This is important because detection and treatment of this recurrent disease can improve the survival and the quality of life of the patient.

The other indication of FDG PET/CT in H&N cancer is in the detection of an unknown primary. This modality should be used when a patient presents with enlarged nodes in the neck and the biopsy shows an epithelial cancer but the primary tumor cannot be found after clinical examination, panendoscopy, CT scan, and possibly MRI scan. The detection and treatment of the primary is important because the treatment of the primary improves the patient's likelihood of success and disease-free survival. We will show you some of the normal patterns seen in the H&N and examples of recurrence detection and detection of the unknown primary.

Top Tip
Sixth most common cancer worldwide
Most occur in tongue base or tonsillar fossa
Strong links to alcohol and tobacco
Treatment may involve surgery, radiotherapy, chemo-
    therapy, or a combination of therapies.

ROLE OF PET/CT IN HEAD AND NECK CANCER

Staging primary head and neck cancer
Identifying sites of recurrence
Distinguishing postoperative change from residual
    disease
Finding the site of an unknown primary tumor
Assessing the response to therapy
Acting as a prognostic tool

NORMAL PATTERNS OF FDG UPTAKE IN THE HEAD AND NECK

In Figure 6.1, the usual axial display of the PET/CT is seen. The CT is displayed on the top left image, the PET is displayed on the top right image, and on the bottom left image, the PET is displayed as a blue-gold distribution that is coregistered with the CT. This final image brings together the anatomical and functional information. This image is at the level of the orbits, and the eyeballs can be seen anteriorly. Here FDG uptake can be seen in both the medial rectus muscles (black arrows) and the lateral rectus muscles (black arrow heads). These muscles are fast twitch glucose dependent muscles and uptake of FDG (as a glucose analogue) is always seen in these muscles. Note that the uptake in the medial rectus is slightly higher than in the medial rectus because of the accommodation of the eyes. FDG uptake is also seen in the grey matter of the brain, at this level in the ante-

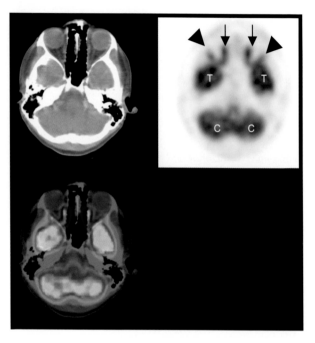

FIGURE 6.1. Normal patterns in the head and neck on PET/CT.

rior temporal lobes (white letter T), and also in the cerebellum
(white letter C). Further uptake is seen in the pons. Constant
blood glucose levels are essential since this is the only energy
substrate that can be used by the brain and therefore high FDG
uptake is always seen in the grey matter.

Figure 6.2 is made at the level of the nasopharynx. Note the
air, black on the CT, in the nasal cavity, and in the right and left
maxillary sinus. The black arrows point at the pair of anterior
depressions in the nasopharynx. This is the torus tubarius and is
the opening of the Eustachian tube into the nasopharynx. Behind
the torus are two further depressions called the fossa of Rosenmueller, or the pharyngeal recesses. This shows normal FDG
uptake (see the blue arrows on the coregistered image), but this
can be much more prominent than in this example. This is
important because it is the most common site for nasopharyngeal cancer. Therefore, when assessing the PET/CT, we need to

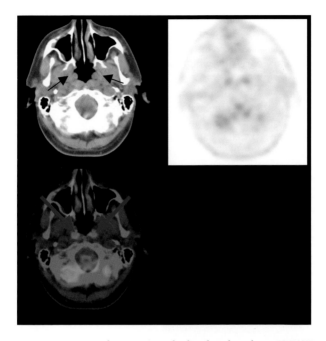

FIGURE 6.2. Normal patterns in the head and neck on PET/CT.

examine this region very closely. Note some uptake in the brain stem that is also normal.

Figure 6.3 is taken just at the level of the oropharynx, and the uvula can clearly be seen at the posterior aspect of the tongue. On the PET, a "double-U"-shape can be seen around the alveolar processes of the maxillary bones on both sides. See the pattern between the two arrows. The FDG appears to out line a horse-shoe shape. Just at the ends of the horseshoe shape are two focal areas of FDG uptake (black arrowheads) which is the uptake seen in the superior aspect of the right and the left palatine tonsil. Uptake of FDG in the tonsils is normal.

Figure 6.4 is taken at the level of the base of the tongue. An inverted V-shape of increased FDG is seen just on the inside of the mandible (black arrows) and this is activity seen in the myolohyoid muscle. This represents glucose use by this muscle elevating the hyoid bone and opening the pharynx to maintain an unconscious open airway during supine resting. FDG uptake is also seen in the lingual tonsil (black arrowheads), which is normal. This is a common place for base of tongue tumors and, just as the fossa of Rosenmueller in the nasopharynx, it must be assessed very carefully when looking at PET/CT of the head and neck.

Because of the complex patterns illustrated and the difficulty in interpretation, some centers routinely administer oral diazepam before the injection of FDG to help prevent unwanted uptake in neck muscles as a result of tension. The diazepam can also decrease the level of physiological brown fat uptake found in some patients. Patients are advised not to talk during the uptake period, as this will result in vocal cord uptake which could be misinterpreted as pathological. Patients are also advised not to move or chew during the uptake phase. Examples of normal and abnormal vocal cord uptake as well as physiological uptake due to muscular tension are found in Chapter 9.

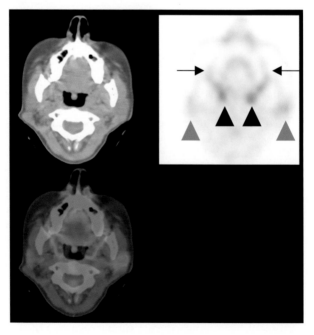

FIGURE 6.3. Normal patterns in the head and neck on PET/CT.

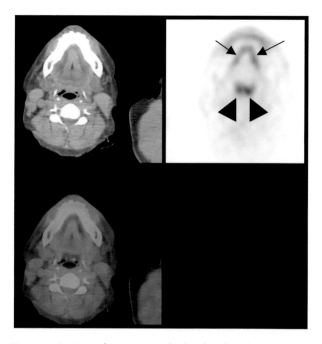

FIGURE 6.4. Normal patterns in the head and neck on PET/CT.

ASSESSMENT
T-Stage Assessment
The combination of PET and CT leads to a very high detection rate of the primary tumor. Recent studies indicate that more than 95% of head and neck cancers will be detected by PET/CT. There may be a reduction in specificity because of complex normal patterns of uptake and in areas of postoperative inflammatory change. PET/CT is excellent in defining the extent of tumor involvement, but the system resolution means that it will under-estimate both submucosal and mucosal spread.

N-Stage Assessment
There are approximately 800 nodes in the body, more 300 of which are found in the head and neck. It is clear that nodal size alone has not been a good discriminator in the assessment of possible malignant involvement. Small nodes can harbor a metastatic tumor and large nodes may simply reflect reactive change.

PET/CT has been shown to be more sensitive than MRI and twice as effective as CT in the detection of nodal metastases. The evaluation of nodal uptake is size dependant, with sensitivity dropping off with decreasing nodal size. With modern combined PET/CT scanners, lesions as small as a few millimeters are demonstrated on the fused PET/CT image. PET/CT will also detect occult disease in approximately 7% of cases.

M-Stage Assessment
PET/CT has had a strong impact in the detection of metastatic lesions with more than 10% of cases demonstrating unexpected occult metastases that were not detected by conventional staging methods. The sensitivity and specificity of metastatic detection are more than 95% and 90% respectively.

DETECTION
Synchronous Primary Disease
As indicated earlier, the etiological affect of alcohol and tobacco have a strong synergistic effect. A heavy smoker has a sevenfold risk of oropharyngeal cancer when compared to a teetotaling, nonsmoker and a thirty seven-fold greater risk if he/she is also a heaver drinker. Synchronous lesions are detected in nearly 20% of patients; they form at a rate of approximately 5% per year. PET/CT often detects lesions that have not even been suspected and some that are not seen with conventional imaging.

An Unknown Pimary Site
PET/CT is useful in those cases where malignant nodes have been detected but conventional work-up has failed to demonstrate a primary site of disease. Approximately 1 in 20 cases present in this way. The early identification and treatment of the primary is associated with improved survival. Studies have shown that PET/CT can detect the primary site in 20 to 50% of such cases. The common sites for false-negative PET/CT scans are often the lingual and palatine tonsils. These are sites of normal physiological uptake and careful note must be made of any asymmetric uptake that can then be visualized directly.

RESPONSE TO THERAPY/DETECTION OF RESIDUAL DISEASE
There is increasing evidence that PET/CT can be used to assess the response of a lesion to radiotherapy or chemotherapy. The standardized uptake value (SUV) is measured both pretherapy and posttherapy. If there has been a significant reduction in SUV as a result of therapy, it is assumed that the metabolic change is

as a result of tumor response. Debate exists as to when post-therapy scans should be carried out and what SUV correlates with long-term response. In general, posttherapy responses to chemotherapy can be carried out quite early–within several weeks. Radiotherapy responses can be assessed as early as three weeks posttherapy, and responses appear to relate to long-term prognosis even though false-positive results can occur at this stage because of radiotherapy-induced inflammatory change.

Some studies suggest that posttherapy FDG uptake with a maximum SUV of 3 or less and those patients who have shown a reduction of over 80% from the pretherapy scan both correlate with a better long-term outcome. More data is required to find the definitive role (if there is one) of the SUV in such circumstances.

PET/CT is extremely sensitive in the detection of residual disease and is also specific if a suitable period of time has elapsed to allow the effects of postoperative change and chemolradio-therapy to diminish. In general, waiting until at least four months after surgery is considered more reliable in detecting residual or recurrent disease. This is extremely important as it has been shown that resection of small volume recurrence equates with an improved survival and quality-of-life benefit.

By six months posttherapy, a normal PET/CT has a very high negative predictive value in out ruling residual disease. However the role of PET/CT in disease surveillance has yet to be clearly defined. Who should we scan and at what interval need to be studied further.

> **Top Tip**
> PET/CT
> Increases the specificity of T stage
> Improves N stage detection
> Improves detection of synchronous disease
> Increased detection of occult metastases
> Is the best non-invasive method for detection of recur-rence/residual disease
> Has a role in assessing response to therapy

Case 1
The figure for Case 1 (see Figure 6.5) show the maximum inten-sity projection (MIP) on the left side and the more familiar axial PET/CT images on the right. The MIP can be considered as a

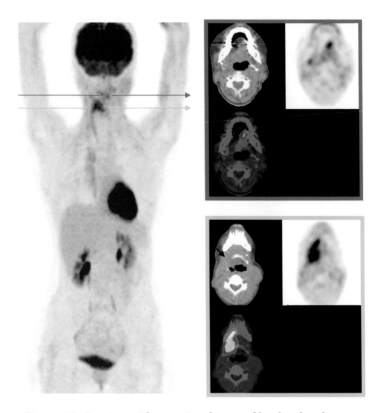

FIGURE 6.5. A patient with a previous history of head and neck cancer.

"glass body" view showing where the FDG goes after it has been injected. See that most of the FDG injected goes to the brain, as described previously. The uptake in the heart is normal and is very variable and activity is also seen being excreted in the urine.

This patient had a history of a tongue tumor and after surgery had a flap reconstruction of the tongue. The patient presented with some pain and a palpable lump at the border of the native tongue and the flap reconstruction. Only the nodule was suspicious clinically and a PET/CT was performed to assess the degree of recurrent disease.

The position of the slice of the axial PET/CT at the level of the palpable nodule is given by the red arrow across the MIP. The gap in the arrow shows you the FDG uptake in the nodule, and this FDG uptake can be seen in the PET/CT images (red box).

This lesion was biopsied and contained only granulation tissue and no tumor.

More extensive FDG uptake is seen deep to the flap reconstruction of the tongue indicated by the yellow arrow, and the gap shows the increased abnormal activity. This recurrent disease was not palpable clinically, and this is often the case deep to flap reconstructions. Also note on the PET/CT coregistered image that the FDG uptake (golden color) extends into the bone of the mandible and that there is destruction of the right side of the hyoid bone (black arrow). Compare this with the normal hyoid bone on the left side. This would indicate advanced recurrent disease that will be very difficult to treat surgically.

Case 2

In Figure 6.6 we have kept the same display with the MIP or "glass body" view showing where the FDG has gone in the patient's body. The red arrow indicates the level of the red boxed axial PET/CT image and the yellow arrow the yellow boxed PET/CT image.

Note at the red level the increased uptake in the left base of the tongue. On the CT, excess soft tissue can also be seen at this level. You can compare this with the other side. Note the normal activity seen in the right lingual tonsil, as discussed earlier. This is the site of the clinically impalpable base of the tongue tumor that was not seen at panendoscopy. The image just below this level also illustrates the primary tumor, but it also shows FDG uptake in a small left-sided node. The FDG uptake can be seen at the black arrow. The small high density node can be seen on the CT at this site (white arrow) and the coregistered image shows FDG uptake at the site of the small node (golden arrow). Note that FDG PET/CT is not reliable in the assessment of nodal spread of H&N tumors.

Case 3

This is the case of a middle-aged man who presented with a swelling involving the right side of his neck. The patient was otherwise quite well but did complain of vague back pain. The neck nodes were biopsied and found to contain metastatic squamous cell carcinoma. Conventional CT and MRI of the head, neck and chest did not reveal the primary lesion. A PET/CT scan was performed in an attempt to identify the primary lesion.

Figure 6.7 is the MIP image. It reveals abnormal uptake within the right side of the neck. Further abnormal uptake is

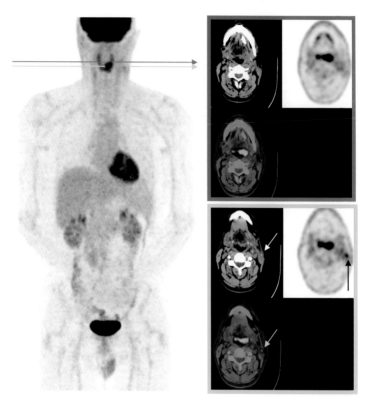

FIGURE 6.6. A right sided neck node removed surgically showed squamous cell cancer, but no primary site was detected.

also visualized in the mediastinum, around the right hilum and in the upper lumbar vertebrae. The axial view through the neck (Figure 6.8 identifies the FDG avid right-sided neck nodes). Figure 6.9 is an axial view through the upper mediastinum that demonstrates a metastatic deposit in the right side of the sternum. No associated bony lesion is seen on the CT component of the study. Figure 6.10 reveals the primary lesion in the right hilum. Bronchoscopy and biopsy later showed this to be a small squamous cell primary. This would have been staged as a T1 lesion on the basis of the lung findings only. Figures 6.11 to 6.13 are the axial, sagittal, and coronal views trough the L2 vertebral metastases. This case has clearly demonstrates the use of PET/CT in the identification of the unknown primary.

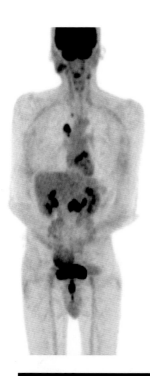

FIGURE 6.7. MIP whole body image showing abnormal uptake in the neck, mediastinum, and lower thoracic vertebrae.

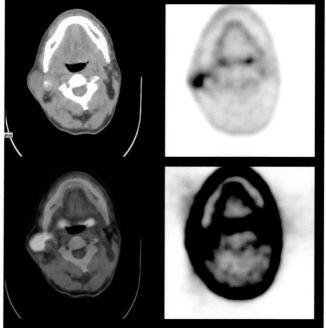

FIGURE 6.8. Abnormal FDG uptake in right neck nodes.

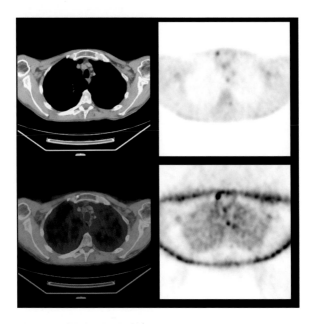

FIGURE 6.9. Axial view through the upper mediastinum reveals a small bony metastatic deposit in the sternum on the right side.

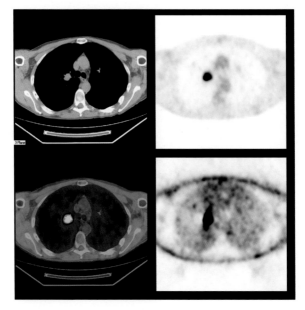

FIGURE 6.10. The abnormal uptake is within the right lung hilum.

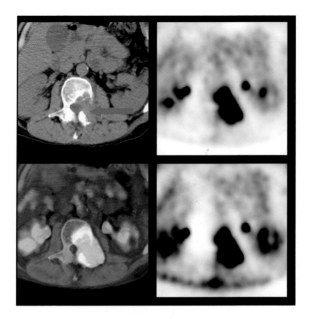

FIGURE 6.11. Axial view through the upper lumbar FDG focus. The CT shows a large, soft tissue mass causing destruction of the posterior vertebral body, as the left lamina and pedicle.

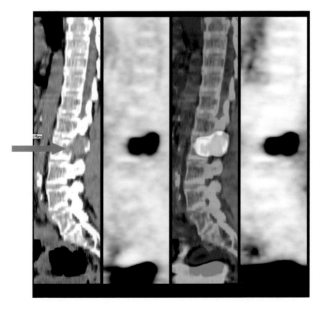

FIGURE 6.12. Sagittal view through the upper lumber FDG focus. The CT shows a lare soft tissue mass causing destruction of the posterior vertebral body, as the left lamina and pedicle.

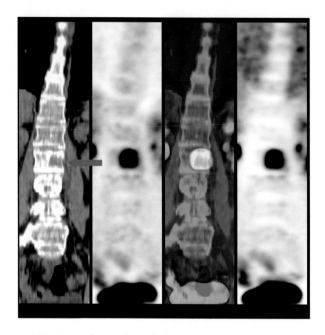

FIGURE 6.13. Coronal view through the upper lumbar FDG focus. The CT shows a large soft tissue mass causing destruction of the posterior vertebral body, as the left lamina and pedicle.

Case 4

This patient has a known squamous cell cancer of the upper third of the oesophagus. The patient had a long history of significant alcohol and tobacco consumption. The patient herself had reported recent onset of hoarseness and worsening dysphagia.

A PET/CT was carried out prior to esophageal surgery. Figure 6.14 is the MIP image which reveals intense upper esophageal FDG uptake as is often found in such cases (red arrow). There is also abnormal uptake in the right side of the upper neck as indicated by the black arrows. Figure 6.15 is an axial view through the upper mediastinum. This image reveals the metabolically active thickened esophagus (red arrow) compressing the upper trachea into a cresentic shape (yellow arrow). Figure 6.16 is a sagittal view through the midline revealing the craniocaudal extent of the esophageal tumor. Figure 6.17 reveals asymmetric FDG uptake within the right vocal cord, best seen on the fused image. There is little or no abnormality found on the CT com-

FIGURE 6.14. MIP image.

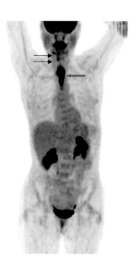

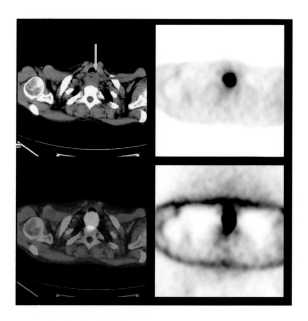

FIGURE 6.15. Axial view through the upper mediastinum.

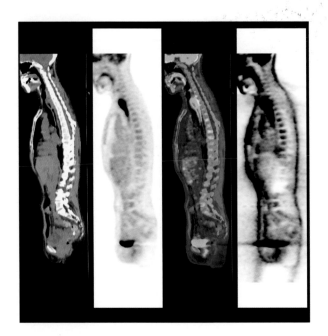

FIGURE 6.16. Sagittal view through the midline.

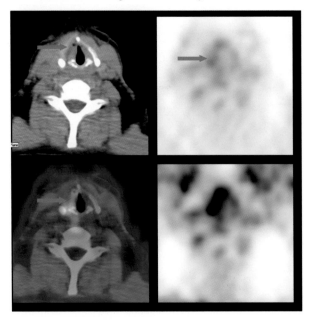

FIGURE 6.17. Asymmetric FDG uptake in the right vocal cord.

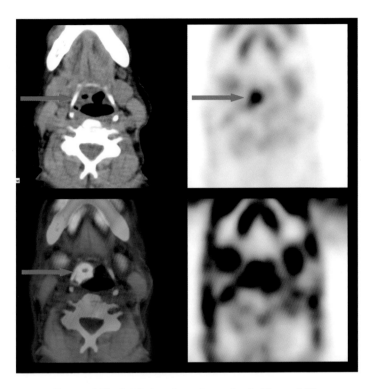

FIGURE 6.18. Axial view 2 cm above that in Figure 6.15.

ponent of the study. Figure 6.18 is another axial view 2 cm above that shown in Figure 6.15. This shows some FDG avid asymmetric thickening at the level of the right superior aryepiglottic fold. Red arrows point to the relevant areas. Direct visualization and biopsy confirmed the presence of a synchronous laryngeal glottic primary, with extension superiorly toward the aryepiglottic fold on the right.

Chapter 7
Melanoma

INTRODUCTION

It may come as a surprise to find that skin cancer is the most common cancer in the world. Skin is the body's largest organ and is directly exposed to external pathogens on a daily basis. Many factors have been implicated in the development of skin cancer, not least the effect of ultraviolet radiation from the sun.

Skin Cancer Types
Basal cell carcinoma 75%
Squamous cell carcinoma 10%
Malignant melanoma 5%

Although malignant melanoma only accounts for approximately 5% of all skin cancers, it is responsible for more than 85% of all skin cancer deaths. The staging systems commonly used for malignant melanoma are outlined later in this chapter, but suffice it to say that small thin localized lesions can often be cured by wide local surgical excision. Thicker lesions growing deeper into the skin are more likely to recur locally or to spread to regional or distant lymph nodes. Distant metastatic spread is generally treated with systemic therapy and has a poor survival rate.

Top Tip
Treatment options are limited and the best hope of a cure is the complete surgical excision of the tumor.

Malignant melanoma shows a strong propensity to spread through the lymphatic system, with metastases often found in distant nodes, lung, liver, brain, bone, and other visceral sites. The pattern of spreading is extremely variable, and unexpected sites of distant disease are commonly found. Unfortunately, in many patients, small metastatic sites do not declare themselves until after the patient has had surgery. In some cases, the surgery involves a wide local excision and lymph node dissection.

Case I

This patient has a histological diagnosis of a T4b primary tumor of the upper back.

Figure 7.1 is the maximum intensity profile whole body image. Conventional imaging revealed a small mediastinal node that was felt to be normal by size criteria. The PET/CT scan demonstrates diffuse intense FDG uptake throughout the liver and a metabolically active mediastinal node. In addition bilateral femoral osseous metastases are identified. Figures 7.2 to 7.4 show the lesions in an axial view and illustrate why these lesions are so hard to detect given the normal appearances on the CT scan. Lesions are indicated by red arrows.

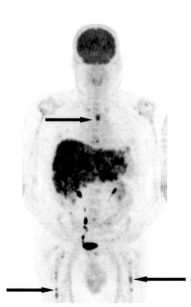

FIGURE 7.1. Melanoma with diffuse liver mets. Further bilateral femoral and mediastinal nodal secondaries.

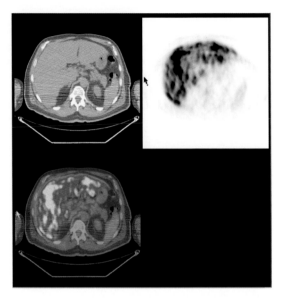

FIGURE 7.2. Melanoma with diffuse liver mets. Normal CT scan appearance.

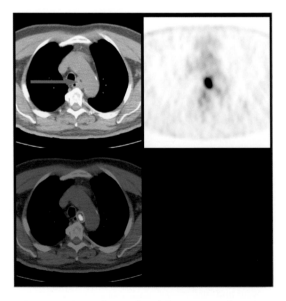

FIGURE 7.3. Mediastinal nodal metastatic deposit.

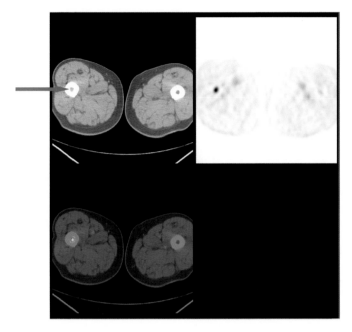

FIGURE 7.4. Melanoma with diffuse liver mets. Further bilateral femoral and mediastinal nodal secondaries.

As with many other tumors it is essential to have a reliable and reproducible system that allows determination of prognosis and the formulation of an appropriate management plan. The possible involvement of regional nodes can be assessed before or at the time of surgery using sentinel node imaging. This is carried out by injecting a radioactive colloid in or around the primary tumor and imaging the subsequent movement of the radioactive tracer into the draining nodes of the tumor.

If the first draining node (the sentinel node) is histologically sampled and does not contain malignant cells, the risk of nodal spread is very low. If the sentinel node does contain metastatic tumor, then radical surgical excision of the regional nodes may result in cure.

Melanoma is generally associated with intense FDG uptake indicating the marked metabolic activity within both the primary tumor and its metastases. PET/CT has been shown to be the single most effective imaging tool in the M staging of malignant melanoma. Because the spread of melanoma is so unpredictable, a whole body PET/CT scan is performed (from vertex to toes).

Case 2

This patient has confirmed recurrent melanoma in the left axillary nodes.

Figure 7.5 is a maximum intensity profile (MIP) image. Multiple foci of increased FDG uptake are seen correlating with metastases in the liver and small bowel. Further lesions are seen along the left and right lateral chest walls. None of these lesions were detected using conventional imaging. Figures 7.6 to 7.9 are images through various lesions found in this patient. Figure 7.6 shows a small left lateral chest wall nodule with intense uptake. Figure 7.7 reveals two unsuspected liver metastases.

Figure 7.8 is the MIP image of the patient's lower limbs revealing an unsuspected right femoral cortical deposit. Figure 7.9 is the axial view through this lesion. Notice the marked

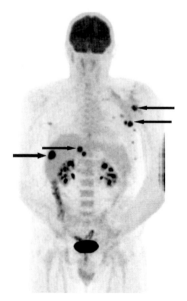

FIGURE 7.5. Recurrent disease demonstrated within the left axilla. No other abnormality detected on CT of chest, abdomen, and pelvis.

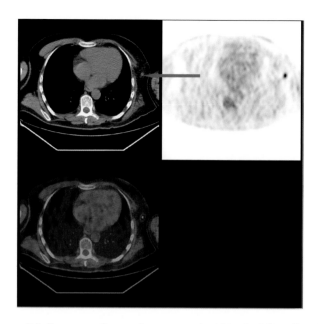

FIGURE 7.6. Recurrent disease demonstrated within the left axilla. This small node was not considered suspicious on CT.

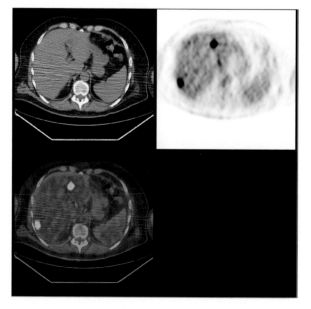

FIGURE 7.7. Two liver metastases with normal CT findings.

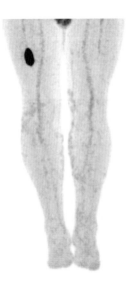

Figure 7.8. Femoral cortical metastatic deposit.

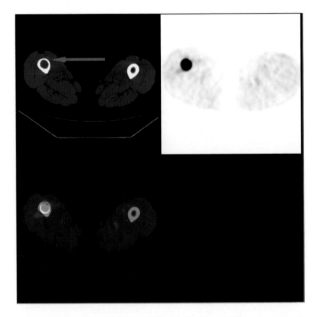

Figure 7.9. Notice the thinning of the right femoral bone cortex (arrow) in comparison to the normal left femoral bone.

cortical thinning as a result of the expanding lesion. Compare this with the normal left cortical thickness. Normal conventional imaging does not extend below the pelvis unless there are specific indications for doing so.

THE ROLE OF PET/CT IN MALIGNANT MELANOMA

The T staging of a primary melanoma is carried out histologically. It often follows a wide local excision or excision biopsy. Most authorities agree that PET/CT has little or no role in the T staging of melanoma. The FDG uptake in small local nodes closely applied to the primary lesion may not be distinguishable from the primary because of the resolution limitations of the detector system. As a result, PET/CT may not be accurate for the N staging of local nodes. PET/CT is, however, extremely useful for the assessment of distant metastatic disease. When PET/CT is used for M staging the overall sensitivities and specificities are more than 90% compared with approximately 50% for conventional staging with CT.

As indicated, involvement of regional nodes and to a greater extent distal nodal involvement is well assessed by PET but the pick-up rate is related directly to the size of the lesion involved. Metastatic melanoma deposits greater than 10 mm in diameter are almost all detected using PET/CT, whereas only 80% of lesions between 6 and 10 mm are found. Lesions with diameters of less than 5 mm are only detected in only just over 20% of cases. Even though the detection of very small lesions is difficult, this is a problem encountered by all imaging modalities.

> **Top Tip**
> Almost all melanoma metastases greater than 1 cm in diameter are detected by PET/CT.

Some studies have shown PET/CT to be approximately twice as accurate as CT in the nodal and distant staging of malignant melanoma. This has resulted in an approximately 30 to 50% management change and the avoidance of unnecessary surgery in approximately 10 to 20%. In particular, PET/CT has been shown to be cost effective in the management of those patients at high risk of metastases. In general clinical stage III and IV (those with nodal or distant metastases), as well as clinically suspicious stage II (T3b), patients are felt to be most suitable for staging with PET/CT.

Patients shown to have regional nodal metastases or isolated distant metastases can be considered for potentially curative surgery, with possible postoperative adjuvant therapy. In patients with more generalized systemic metastases, discussion can take place on strategies for systemic therapy disseminated disease, in a cost-effective way without recourse to further diagnostic procedures.

Case 3

Although PET/CT is recommended for higher stage lesions, it is possible to detect small T1 lesions if they have sufficient uptake. Figure 7.10 is the lateral MIP of a patient who was having a scan to assess response to chemotherapy for non-Hodgkin's lymphoma. The image reveals a tiny intense focus of uptake lying

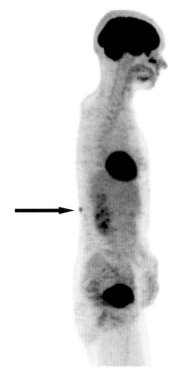

FIGURE 7.10. Lateral MIP view with a small focus of uptake posteriorly (arrow).

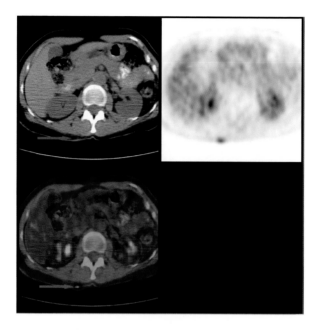

FIGURE 7.11. Axial PET/CT with a small focus of uptake posteriorly (arrow).

superficially. The PET/CT (Figure 7.11) reveals a tiny soft tissue distortion barely discernable on the scan. This had not been previously noticed but a small lesion was found on clinical examination which was histologically confirmed as a T1 malignant melanoma.

Top Tip

PET/CT is twice as accurate as CT in the detection of distant disease.

PET/CT avoids unnecessary surgery and results in significant management change.

PET/CT is best employed in patients with suspected nodal or distant metastatic involvement, or a high risk of such spread.

PET/CT can also be employed in restaging patients before the removal of presumed solitary metastases or in the confirmation of recurrent disease. The use of PET/CT in the assessment of treatment response and in surveillance for relapse has shown promise, but it is not yet widely practiced.

Case 4
This patient had an excision biopsy of a malignant melanoma of the right forearm. A staging CT scan revealed a small right supraclavicular node, which was felt to represent a solitary metastatic lesion. The patient had a PET/CT scan (Figure 7.12). The MIP image clearly reveals two abnormal foci of increased uptake in

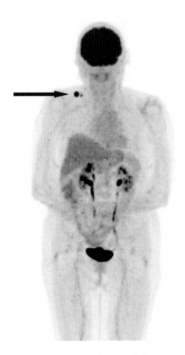

FIGURE 7.12. Right supraclavicular nodal metastases from a right forearm primary.

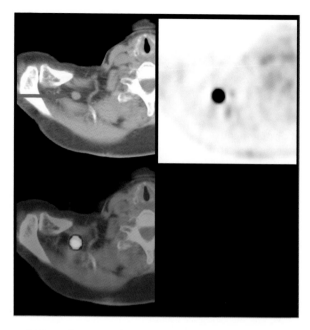

FIGURE 7.13. Right supraclavicular nodal metastases from a right forearm primary.

the right supraclavicular fossa. Figure 7.13 is the corresponding axial image through this level. Two small intensely active supraclavicular nodes are present. These were excised and confirmed to be metastatic melanoma.

Areas Where PET/CT May Prove Useful in Malignant Melanoma

In maglignant melanoma, PET/CT is most useful in:

1. Staging of patients with suspected nodal or distant metastatic involvement or a high risk of such spread.
2. Staging of suspicious lesions at presentation.
3. Restaging patients prior to surgical metastectomy.
4. Confirmation of suspected recurrence.

PET/CT has a possible, but as yet unproven, role in:
1. Monitoring the response to therapy.
2. Disease surveillance.

Top Tip
PET/CT can stage melanoma with a higher diagnostic accuracy than any other noninterventional method. This can result in significant stage and management change.

Case 5

This final case again illustrates the difficulty that conventional imaging can present in detecting and determining the extent of melanoma spread. This patient had a recurrent melanoma of the groin and unsuspected metastases to the lower limbs.

Figure 7.14 is the axial view through the upper groin level. This reveals a small active node in the right groin which on

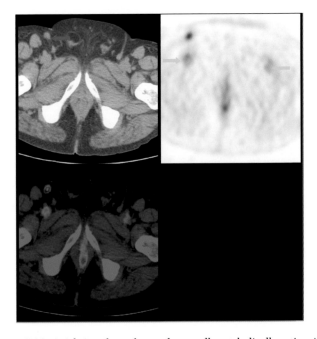

FIGURE 7.14. Axial view through reveals a small metabolically active right groin recurrence. The red arrow on the CT scan points to the active right groin node, and the yellow arrows on the PET scan point to blood pool activity within the fermoral vessels.

FIGURE 7.15. Unsuspected lower limb metastases.

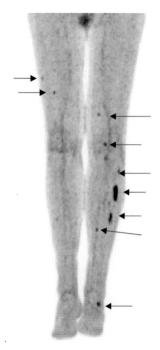

biopsy was confirmed as recurrent disease. Figure 7.15 is the MIP view of the lower limbs demonstrating multiple bilateral metastases that were not suspected following conventional imaging. Figures 7.16 and 7.17 are coronal and axial views through the lower limbs revealing the lesions to lie within the muscles of the leg.

The PET/CT criteria for assessing response to therapy is still under debate and requires further research, but it is certainly related to a marked decrease in the SUV between the pretherapy and posttherapy scans. The role of PETCT in follow-up surveillance and the interval between surveillance scans is also unresolved, but many authorities propose that annual PET/CT imaging is appropriate. In our experience, this degree of frequency will result in many interval relapses occurring between scans. More frequent scanning would however place an intolerable burden on scarce resources and would require an evidence base to justify the approach.

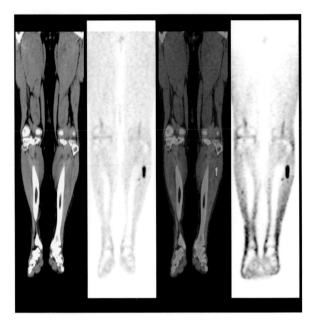

FIGURE 7.16. Coronal view showing some of the active soft tissue metastases.

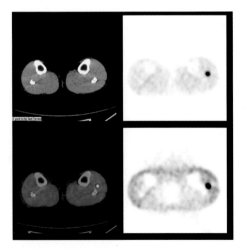

FIGURE 7.17. Axial view shows one of the metastatic deposits within the soft tissue muscles of the left calf. No CT abnormality is found.

STAGING, TREATMENT AND PROGNOSIS

Accurate staging of the extent of the disease is essential to determine the prognosis and to guide management strategy. Clark and Breslow clearly demonstrated that the extent of the invasion of the melanoma into the skin was the most accurate method of predicting the risk of relapse and the outcome. Clark related the depth of invasion to the penetration of the histologically defined layers of the skin, whereas Breslow measured the thickness of the tumor in millimeters. In the most recent TNM staging classification, the Breslow thickness is used almost exclusively in preference to the Clark level for determination of T stage. In additional, the presence of tumor ulceration on histology is included as a determinant of T staging (see Table 7.1).

The suffix "a" is added if there is no ulceration on histological examination. The suffix "b" is added if ulceration is present or, for T1 tumors only, the suffix "b" is also added for Clark level 4 or 5 invasion.

Clinical stages I and II are confined to those patients who have no evidence of regional or distant metastases (any T stage, N0, M0). If there is regional spread to either lymph nodes or to lymphatics (satellite or in-transit metastases), this will be recorded in the N stage (N1 to N3) and will be classified as clinical Stage III disease. Distant metastases will be included in the M stage category as M1 and represent Stage IV disease.

Stages I and II melanoma are considered to represent localized disease only; stage 3 involves metastases to the regional draining nodes; stage 4 exists if there is evidence of distant metastatic spread to skin or lymph nodes (see Table 7.2).

Disease management is shown in Table 7.3. Stage I to III tumors are managed by complete surgical excision with appropriate margins and follow-up. This represents the only realistic prospect of long-term survival. Adjuvant therapy for high-risk patients using a one-year regimen of high dose adjuvant interferon improves disease-free survival, but it is of uncertain benefit to long-term survival and is associated with considerable short-term morbidity.

For Stage IV patients it is still appropriate to consider complete resection of isolated metastases, if feasible, as this unusual situation can result in long-term cure. Otherwise palliative therapy with chemotherapy or immunotherapy results in modest response rates of 15 to 30%, but with few durable responses. The median survival for patients with stage IV disease is less than one year. For patients with brain, bone, or troublesome soft tissue metastases, radiotherapy can be effective in symptom control.

TABLE 7.1. TNM Classification and Stage Grouping

DEFINITION OF TNM

Patients with melanoma *in situ* are categorized as Tis. Those patients with melanoma presentations that are indeterminate or cannot be microstaged should be categorized as Tx. The T category of melanoma is classified primarily by measuring the thickness of the melanoma as defined by Dr. Alexander Breslow. The T category thresholds of melanoma thickness are defined in whole integers (i.e., at 1.0, 2.0, and 4.0 mm). Melanoma ulceration is the absence of an intact epidermis overlying the primary melanoma, assessed by histopathologic examination.[8–10] The level of invasion, as defined by Dr. Wallace Clark,[11] is used to define subcatagories of T1 melanomas but not for thicker melanomas (i.e., T2, T3, or T4).

Regional metastases most commonly present in the regional lymph nodes. The actual number of nodal metastases identified by the pathologist must be reported for staging purposes. A second staging definition is related to tumor burden: microscopic vs. macroscopic. Thus those patients without clinical or radiologic evidence of lymph node metastases, but who have pathologically documented nodal metastases, are defined by convention as exhibiting "microscopic" or "clinically occult" nodal metastases. In contrast, melanoma patients with both clinical evidence of nodal metastases *and* pathologic examination documenting the number of nodal metastases (after therapeutic lymphadenectomy) are defined by convention as having "macroscopic" or "clinically apparent" nodal metastases. Regional metastases also include intralymphatic metastases, defined as the presence of clinical or microscopic satellites around a primary melanoma, and/or in-transit metastases between the primary melanoma and the regional lymph nodes.

Distant metastases are staged primarily by the organ or site(s) in which they are located. A second factor in staging is the presence or absence of an elevated serum LDH. An elevated serum LDH should be used only when there are two or more determinations obtained more than 24 hours apart, because an elevated serum LDH on a single determination can be falsely positive as a result of hemolysis or other factors unrelated to melanoma metastases.

Primary Tumor (T)

TX	Primary tumor cannot be assessed (e.g., shave biopsy or regressed melanoma)
T0	No evidence of primary tumor
Tis	Melanoma *in situ*
T1	Melanoma ≤1.0 mm in thickness with or without ulceration
T1a	Melanoma ≤1.0 mm in thickness and level II or III, no ulceration
T1b	Melanoma ≤1.0 mm in thickness and level IV or V or with ulceration
T2	Melanoma 1.01–2 mm in thickness with or without ulceration
T2a	Melanoma 1.01–2.0 mm in thickness, no ulceration

TABLE 7.1. *Continued*

T2b	Melanoma 1.01–2.0 mm in thickness, with ulceration
T3	Melanoma 2.01–4 mm in thickness with or without ulceration
T3a	Melanoma 2.01–4 mm in thickness, no ulceration
T3b	Melanoma 2.01–4 mm in thickness, with ulceration
T4	Melanoma greater than 4.0 mm in thickness with or without ulceration
T4a	Melanoma >4.0 mm in thickness, no ulceration
T4b	Melanoma >4.0 mm in thickness, with ulceration

Regional Lymph Nodes (N)

NX	Regional lymph nodes cannot be assessed
N0	No regional lymph node metastasis
N1	Metastasis in one lymph node
N1a	Clinically occult (microscopic) metastasis
N1b	Clinically apparent (macroscopic) metastasis
N2	Metastasis in two to three regional nodes or intralymphatic regional metastasis without nodal metastases
N2a	Clinically occult (microscopic) metastasis
N2b	Clinically apparent (macroscopic) metastasis
N2c	Satellite or in-transit metastasis *without* nodal metastasis
N3	Metastasis in four or more regional nodes, or matted metastatic nodes, or in-transit metastasis or satellite(s) *with* metastasis in regional node(s)

Distant Metastasis (M)

MX	Distant metastasis cannot be assessed
M0	No distant metastasis
M1	Distant metastasis
M1a	Metastasis to skin, subcutaneous tissues or distant lymph nodes
M1b	Metastasis to lung
M1c	Metastasis to all other visceral sites or distant metastasis at any site associated with an elevated serum lactic dehydrogenase (LDH)

STAGE GROUPING

Patients with primary melanomas with no evidence of regional or distant metastases (either clinically or pathologically) are divided into two stages: Stage I for early-stage patients with "low risk" for metastases and melanoma-specific mortality and Stage II for those with "intermediate risk" for metastases and melanoma-specific mortality. There are no substages for clinical Stage III melanoma, because criteria for subgrouping can be inaccurate. Pathologic Stage III patients with regional metastases make up a very heterogeneous group that has been divided into three subgroups according to prognostic risk. Stage IIIA patients have up to three microscopic nodal metastases arising from a non-ulcerating primary melanoma and have an "intermediate risk" for distant metastases and melanoma-specific survival. Stage IIIB patients have up to three

TABLE 7.1. *Continued*

macroscopic nodal metastases arising from a non-ulcerating melanoma, or have up to three microscopic nodal metastases arising from an ulcerating melanoma, or have intralymphatic metastases without nodal metastases. They constitute a "high-risk" group prognostically. The remaining patients are Stage IIIC and are at "very high risk" for distant metastases and melanoma-specific mortality. The presence of melanoma ulceration "up-stages" the prognosis of Stage I, II, and III patients compared to patients with melanomas of equivalent thickness without ulceration or those with nodal metastases arising from a non-ulceration melanoma. There are no subgroups of Stage IV melanoma.

CLINICAL STAGE GROUPING			
Stage 0	Tis	N0	M0
Stage IA	T1a	N0	M0
Stage IB	T1b	N0	M0
	T2a	N0	M0
Stage IIA	T2b	N0	M0
	T3a	N0	M0
Stage IIB	T3b	N0	M0
	T4a	N0	M0
Stage IIC	T4b	N0	M0
Stage III	Any T	N1	M0
	Any T	N2	M0
	Any T	N3	M0
Stage IV	Any T	Any N	M1

Note: Clinical staging includes microstaging of the primary melanoma and clinical/radiological evaluation for metastases. By convention, it should be used after complete excision of the primary melanoma with clinical assessment for regional and distant metastases.

PATHOLOGIC STAGE GROUPING			
Stage 0	Tis	N0	M0
Stage IA	T1a	N0	M0
Stage IB	T1b	N0	M0
	T2a	N0	M0
Stage IIA	T2b	N0	M0
	T3a	N0	M0
Stage IIB	T3b	N0	M0
	T4a	N0	M0
Stage IIC	T4b	N0	M0
Stage IIIA	T1–4a	N1a	M0
	T1–4a	N2a	M0

TABLE 7.1. *Continued*

Stage IIIB	T1–4b	N1a	M0
	T1–4b	N2a	M0
	T1–4a	N1b	M0
	T1–4a	N2b	M0
	T1–4a/b	N2c	M0
Stage IIIC	T1–4b	N1b	M0
	T1–4b	N2b	M0
	Any T	N3	M0
Stage IV	Any T	Any N	M1

Note: Pathologic staging includes microstaging of the primary melanoma and pathologic information about the regional lymph nodes after partial or complete lymphadenectomy. Pathologic Stage 0 or Stage IA patients are the exception; they do not require pathologic evaluation of their lymph nodes.

Source: Used with the permission of the American Joint Committee on Cancer (AJCC), Chicago, Illinois. The original source for this material is the AJCC Cancer Staging Manual, Sixth Edition (2002) published by Springer-New York, www.springeronline.com.

TABLE 7.2. Melanoma Prognosis by Stage

Stage	1	II	III	IV
10-year survival	>80%	60–80%	30–50%	<5%

TABLE 7.3. Disease Management

	Treatment strategy	Prognosis	5-year survival
Basal cell	Excisional surgery or radiotherapy	Excellent	>99%
Squamous cell	Excisional surgery or radiotherapy, with close follow-up for nodal relapse	Good	>90%
Malignant melanoma, localized or regional	Excision +/– adjuvant Immunotherapy, with close follow-up	Moderate	>30%
Malignant melanoma, disseminated	Systemic therapy, (rarely complete excision)	Very poor	<5%

Metastatic melanoma is a fertile area for research with many new chemotherapy, immunotherapy and targeted therapy approaches being explored in clinical trials.

Basal and squamous cell carcinoma are much less deadly and share common characteristics. Unlike malignant melanoma these tumors have effective treatment options (see Table 7.3) and cure rates of more than 90%. PET/CT is not routinely used in the staging of basal or squamous cell cancer of the skin.

Patients with disseminated malignant melanoma have a very poor prognosis, with a median survival of only 12 months. Because lesions are generally radioresistant, the use of radiotherapy is not universally recommended. There are reports of beneficial effects in some peripheral lesions treated with intermittent high dose fractions and occasional improvement in brain, bone, and soft tissue lesions. Chemotherapeutic regimes are generally disappointing, with response rates of only 20 to 30% and few long lasting remissions reported. Immunotherapy with Alpha interferon had been introduced and despite initial encouraging signs has only produced short-lived responses in 10 to 20% of individuals. The relatively recent development of peptide based vaccines has again raised the hope of a long term improvement in the cure rate.

Chapter 8
Cancers of the Male and Female Reproductive Systems

INTRODUCTION

In contrast to many other tumor groups, the role of FDG-PET and PET/CT in gynecological and testicular malignancies is much less clearly defined. There is, however, reliable evidence that FDG-PET does have a useful role in the management of these cancers and, with the introduction of PET/CT, this is likely to advance. FDG-PET experience in gynecological malignancies has, to date, been largely confined to ovarian and cervical carcinoma.

OVARIAN CANCER

Ovarian cancer is associated with late presentation and poor prognosis. At present, the role of FDG-PET has largely been in assessment for recurrent disease and, although the overall numbers reported in the literature are relatively small, the results support the use of FDG-PET. With PET/CT, the investigation is likely to be even more successful, particularly in reducing the number of false-positive reports.

Staging of Disease

There is debate as to the role of PET/CT in initial staging. With surgery considered key in the role of gaining control of tumor burden and the majority of patients receiving adjuvant chemotherapy, PET/CT is not commonly used in preoperative staging. There are currently multicenter trials assessing potential screening modalities for ovarian cancer with view to early detection. If screening for ovarian cancer were to become available, one would anticipate PET/CT becoming an essential tool in patient staging and in directing surgery in earlier, small volume disease. Conventional imaging modalities do not reliably identify small volume disease.

Restaging of Disease

"Second-look" exploratory surgery was originally used in assessment for recurrence, but after studies failed to show any survival benefit, many clinicians have adopted a 'wait-and-see' basis, combined with CT, MRI, U/S and the use of tumor markers—notably Ca125.

Each of these modalities has significant shortcomings in determining disease status. In data reporting the sensitivity and specificity of CT, MRI and U/S in three common sites of metastatic disease, peritoneum, lymph nodes and the liver, none of the three modalities showed sensitivities above 50% in nodal disease, with only ultrasound reporting a sensitivity of >50% in identification of liver lesions. Both CT and MRI identified peritoneal disease with a high degree of sensitivity. Lesions smaller than 2 cm were poorly identified by all modalities. Similarly, while an elevated Ca125 is associated with recurrence in approximately 80% of patients, in up to 33% of patients, recurrent disease is associated with normal Ca125 levels.

The current primary indication for FDG-PET/CT in ovarian cancer is where there is suspicion of recurrent disease, either clinically or, more frequently, where Ca125 is elevated and/or rising but conventional imaging has been negative.

Assessment of Treatment Response

As with the other tumor groups, response to therapy is likely to be an emerging indication, as the number of second-line chemotherapy drugs increases. This is not currently standard practice with many fundamentals (e.g., timing of scans and prognostic benefit have not yet established).

Top Tip
PET/CT enhances detection rates when used as an adjunct to conventional imaging modalities.
Key indication is when elevated/rising CA125 levels with normal CT/MRI.

Issues with Scan Interpretation

Ovarian uptake of FDG is not always pathological. It is seen in relation to ovulatory activity, so a relevant history should always be obtained. Another issue is the limitations in identifying local and early disease.

THE UTERINE CARCINOMAS
In contrast to ovarian cancer, the uterine carcinomas (i.e., endometrium and cervix) tend to present earlier and have much better survival rates. Although studies have shown that FDG does accumulate in endometrial cancers, PET/CT is not currently routinely used in management of these tumors. There is growing evidence that FDG-PET and PET/CT does contribute to patient management in cervical cancers.

CARCINOMA OF THE CERVIX
Both CT and MR are used to stage carcinoma of the cervix. The limitation of this structural staging is often, as is the case for all tumors, the arbitrary 1 cm cut off for differentiation of malignant from benign disease. It is now accepted that small nodes can harbor disease and large nodes may only be reactive. As lymph node staging is fundamental in the management of cervical cancer both in terms of survival and treatment, accurate assessment of nodal involvement is required.

Staging
PET performs particularly well in detection of distant metastases and paraaortic disease, at least as well as CT and MR in pelvic nodal disease, and less well in local disease. This is attributed to the high levels of excreted activity in the bladder. In early disease, FDG-PET outperformed MRI.

Nodal metastases are common and seen in almost 20% of patients with Stage Ib disease (outside cervix, upper two-thirds of the vagina may be involved, but not as far as the pelvic wall) and more than 60% of patients with stage III disease (disease to the pelvic wall and/or lower one-third of the vagina). Given the decreased survival rates associated with paraaortic nodal disease, PET/CT is being increasingly used to assess disease in these nodes.

Case I
This patient had a diagnosis of stage IIa cancer of the cervix, and it was assumed that she had been successfully treated with surgical resection and pelvic lymphadenectomy. A follow up PET/CT scan was performed to assess possible small paraaortic nodal involvement demonstrated on CT. The nodes were not significantly enlarged by conventional size criteria.

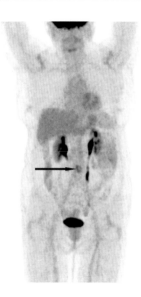

FIGURE 8.1. Low-grade midline FDG uptake.

Figure 8.1 is the whole body MIP that reveals a low-grade focus of FDG uptake in the midline (arrow). Figure 8.2 is an axial view through this low-grade uptake, and it reveals a mesenteric metastatic deposit (arrow). No abnormal nodal uptake was demonstrated within any paraaortic nodes. The referring clinician and surgeon were not convinced of this finding and it was agreed to reimage the patient in six months. A follow-up PET/CT (Figure 8.3) was carried out six months later. It revealed significant disease progression in the interval since the original PET scan. Notice the increased intensity of FDG uptake in the original lesion (arrow) during the six-month interval.

Restaging
FDG-PET has been shown to be superior over conventional imaging in detection of recurrent disease. This is important as further treatment options may be available for those who have relapsed and improved survival rates using FDG-PET for restaging have been reported. PET-CT, particularly where conventional imaging is normal, is likely to be even more beneficial than PET only.

Case 2
This case is a patient with a stage Ib cervical cancer treated with radiotherapy and a PET/CT was carried out to assess response to

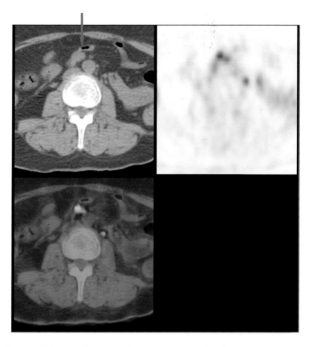

FIGURE 8.2. Axial image demonstrating a focal mesenteric met.

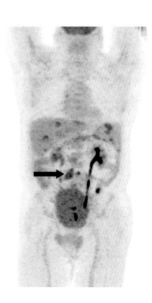

FIGURE 8.3. Multiple sites of peritoneal and hepatic disease.

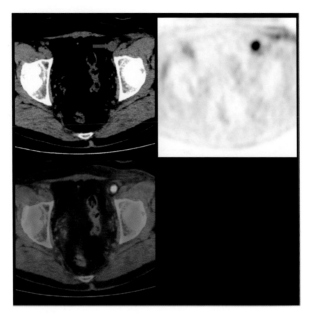

FIGURE 8.4. Left external iliac FDG positive node.

therapy. Figure 8.4 reveals an abnormal left external iliac node with focal FDG uptake. The node was removed and revealed metastatic cells. The patient received further consolidation radiotherapy and underwent pelvic lymphadenectomy.

Treatment Planning
In addition to patients with advanced (Stage III, IV) disease where radiotherapy is the primary treatment, a significant number of patients receive postoperative radiotherapy to the pelvis. Given the paramount importance of determining paraaortic disease status and the superiority of FDG-PET over CT and MRI in assessment of paraaortic disease, PET-CT is being increasingly used to guide therapy planning. If the study is positive, radiotherapy fields will be modified.

Response to Treatment
At present there are no guidelines as to the role of PET in assessing response to treatment.

> **Top Tip**
> Presence/absence of paraaortic disease has high prognostic significance.
> PET/CT "best" imaging modality for paraaortic disease.
> PET/CT outperforms conventional imaging for distant disease.

Issues with Scan Interpretation

The issues with interpreting scans is that the differentiation of physiological ureteric activity from paraaortic nodal disease can be difficult in some cases. In additions, there are limitations in the detection of local disease because of high activity in bladder.

TESTICULAR NEOPLASMS

Most testicular neoplasms (95%) are germ cell tumors. These are subdivided into seminoma and nonseminomatous germ cell tumors (NSGCT). The NSCGCT group includes teratomas of varying degrees of differentiation, tumors containing mixed cell lines of teratomas, and mixed tumors with both teratoma and seminoma components. The division reflects the different treatments and outcomes. The other 5% of testicular neoplasia includes lymphoma, and metastases. This section is confined to germ cell tumors.

Initial management for all germ cell testicular tumors is surgical, with radical inguinal orchidectomy the procedure of choice. The key prognostic markers are histological subtype, tumor extension to the spermatic cord, invasion of local vessels and the serum level of the tumor markers α-fetoprotein (AFP) and human chorionic gonadotrophin-β (HCG).

> **Top Tip**
> Prognostic indicators include:
> Histology
> Tumor extension
> AFP level
> HCG level

Pure seminomas may have a modest elevation of HCG, but AFP levels should be normal. Elevated AFP is seen in about 70% of teratomas, with elevated HCG in about 50% of the cases. These markers reflect different cell lines and accordingly do not necessarily respond in the same way to chemotherapy.

Staging of Disease
With advances in treatment, a growing number of patients will be cured and great emphasis is placed on accurate initial staging. Sensitive assays of tumor markers contribute greatly to staging, as does imaging such as CT and MRI. Both PET and PET/CT provide an increase in conventional diagnostic accuracy. FDG-PET has positive and negative predictive values superior to those reported for conventional imaging in staging, including early disease.

FDG-PET however is not considered a reliable tool for disease evaluation in mature teratoma differentiated (MTD).

Restaging of Disease
PET/CT has positive and negative predictive values superior to those reported for conventional imaging in restaging. This is particularly important in those patients for whom there are no available tumor markers to provide an early and sensitive indication of relapse. PET and now PET/CT also has a key role when tumor markers are rising and conventional imaging has been unrewarding.

Case 3
This case is a patient who had a PET/CT scan to restage disease extent following a rise in tumor markers. He had previously undergone an orchidectomy for a testicular seminoma.

The MIP view (Figure 8.5) shows a focus of uptake in the left hemipelvis which could represent activity within the distal left ureter. The axial view through this focus demonstrate small volume recurrent disease in a small left common iliac node (Figure 8.6).

Treatment Planning
Early stage seminomas have high cure rates associated with surgery and radiotherapy, with more advanced disease showing good response rates to chemotherapy. There is debate about the role of radiotherapy in early disease and, as a significant number of pure seminomas are not associated with abnormal tumor markers, PET/CT may have a role in treatment planning where

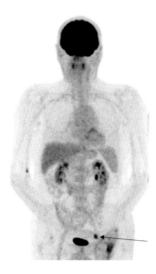

FIGURE 8.5. MIP image demonstrating a left sided pelvic focus of uptake.

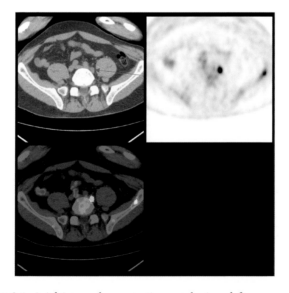

FIGURE 8.6. Axial image demonstrating uptake in a left common iliac node representing recurrent disease.

more conservative treatment of early stage disease (i.e., surgery only is being offered). In NSGCT, chemotherapy is the mainstay of treatment and as such, FDG-PET has not played a significant role in treatment planning.

Assessment of Treatment Response
Structural imaging does not characterize the nature of residual masses or residual lymphadenopathy. FDG-PET and PET/CT allows assessment of metabolic activity still regarded as "abnormal" on conventional imaging.

> **Top Tip**
> High positive predictive value for recurrent disease
> Useful with rising tumor markers and normal CT and/or MRI
> Useful in the assessment of residual lymphadenopathy

Issues with Scan Interpretation
The issues in interpreting scans are that FDG-PET is *not* reliable in MTD and there is difficulty in differentiating physiological ureteric activity from paraaortic nodal disease.

STAGING OF TESTICULAR CANCER

TABLE 8.1. TNM Classification and Stage Grouping

DEFINITION OF TNM

Primary Tumor (T)
The extent of primary tumor is usually classified after radical orchiectomy, and for this reason, a *pathologic* stage is assigned.

*pTX	Primary tumor cannot be assessed
pT0	No evidence of primary tumor (e.g., histologicscar in testis)
pTis	Intratubular germ cell neoplasia (carcinoma *in situ*)
PT1	Tumor limited to the testis and epididymis without vascular/lymphatic invasion; tumor may invade into the tunica albuginea but not the tunica vaginalis
pT2	Tumor limited to the testis and epididymis with vascular/lymphatic invasion, or tumor extending through the tunica albuginea with involvement of the tunica vaginalis
PT3	Tumor invades the spermatic cord with or without vascular/lymphatic invasion
pT4	Tumor invades the scrotum with or without vascular/lymphatic invasion

TABLE 8.1. *Continued*

Note: Except for pTis and pT4, extent of primary tumor is classified by radical orchiectomy. TX may be used for other categories in the absence of radical orchiectomy.

Regional Lymph Nodes (N)

Clinical

NX   Regional lymph nodes cannot be assessed
N0   No regional lymph node metastasis
N1   Metastasis with a lymph node mass 2 cm or less in greatest dimension; or multiple lymph nodes, none more than 2 cm in greatest dimension
N2   Metastasis with a lymph node mass more than 2 cm but not more than 5 cm in greatest dimension; or multiple lymph nodes, any one mass greater than 2 cm but not more than 5 cm in greatest dimension
N3   Metastasis with a lymph node mass more than 5 cm in greatest dimension

Pathologic (pN)

pNX   Regional lymph nodes cannot be assessed
pN0   No regional lymph node metastasis
pN1   Metastasis with a lymph node mass 2 cm or less in greatest dimension and less than or equal to 5 nodes positive, none more than 2 cm in greatest dimension
pN2   Metastasis with a lymph node mass more than 2 cm but not more than 5 cm in greatest dimension; or more than 5 nodes positive, none more than 5 cm; or evidence of extranodal extension of tumor
pN3   Metastasis with a lymph node mass more than 5 cm in greatest dimension

Distant Metastasis (M)

MX   Distant metastasis cannot be assessed
M0   No distant metastasis
M1   Distant metastasis
M1a   Non-regional nodal or pulmonary metastasis
M1b   Distant metastasis other than to non-regional lymph nodes and lungs

Serum Tumor Markers (S)

SX   Marker studies not available or not performed
S0   Marker study levels within normal limits
S1   LDH $< 1.5 \times$ N* **AND**
       hCG (mIu/ml) < 5000 **AND**
       AFP (ng/ml) < 1000
S2   LDH $1.5–10 \times$ N **OR**
       hCG (mIu/ml) 5000–50,000 **OR**
       AFP (ng/ml) 1000–10,000

TABLE 8.1. *Continued*

S3	LDH > 10 × N **OR**
	hCG (mIu/ml) > 50,000 **OR**
	AFP (ng/ml) > 10,000

*N indicates the upper limit of normal for the LDH assay.

STAGE GROUPING

Stage 0	pTis	N0	M0	S0
Stage I	pT1–4	N0	M0	SX
Stage IA	pT1	N0	M0	S0
Stage IB	pT2	N0	M0	S0
	pT3	N0	M0	S0
	pT4	N0	M0	S0
Stage IS	Any pT/Tx	N0	M0	S1–3
Stage II	Any pT/Tx	N1–3	M0	SX
Stage IIA	Any pT/Tx	N1	M0	S0
	Any pT/Tx	N1	M0	S1
Stage IIB	Any pT/Tx	N2	M0	S0
	Any pT/Tx	N2	M0	S1
Stage IIC	Any pT/Tx	N3	M0	S0
	Any pT/Tx	N3	M0	S1
Stage III	Any pT/Tx	Any N	M1	SX
Stage IIIA	Any pT/Tx	Any N	M1a	S0
	Any pT/Tx	Any N	M1a	S1
Stage IIIB	Any pT/Tx	N1–3	M0	S2
	Any pT/Tx	Any N	M1a	S2
Stage IIIC	Any pT/Tx	N1–3	M0	S3
	Any pT/Tx	Any N	M1a	S3
	Any pT/Tx	Any N	M1b	Any S

Source: Used with the permission of the American Joint Committee on Cancer (AJCC), Chicago, Illinois. The original source for this material is the AJCC Cancer Staging Manual, Sixth Edition (2002) published by Springer-New York, www.springeronline.com.

TABLE 8.2. TNM Classification and Stage Grouping

DEFINITION OF TNM

The definitions of the T categories correspond to the stages accepted by FIGO. FIGO stages are further subdivided by histologic grade of tumor—for example, Stage IC G2. Both systems are included for comparison.

Primary Tumor (T) (Surgical-Pathologic findings)

TNM Categories	FIGO Stages	
TX		Primary tumor cannot be assessed
T0		No evidence of primary tumor

TABLE 8.2. *Continued*

Tis	0	Carcinoma *in situ*
T1	I	Tumor confined to corpus uteri
T1a	IA	Tumor limited to endometrium
T1b	IB	Tumor invades less than one-half of the myometrium
T1c	IC	Tumor invades one-half or more of the myometrium
T2	II	Tumor invades cervix but does not extend beyond uterus
T2a	IIA	Tumor limited to the glandular epithelium of the endocervix. There is no evidence of connective tissue stromal invasion
T2b	IIB	Invasion of the stromal connective tissue of the cervix
T3	III	Local and/or regional spread as defined below
T3a	IIIA	Tumor involves serosa and/or adnexa (direct extension or metastasis) and/or cancer cells in ascites or peritoneal washings
T3b	IIIB	Vaginal involvement (direct extension or metastasis)
T4	IVA	Tumor invades bladder mucosa and/or bowel mucosa (bullous edema is not sufficient to classify a tumor asT4)

Regional Lymph Nodes (N)

NX		Regional lymph nodes cannot be assessed
N0		No regional lymph node metastasis
N1	IIIC	Regional lymph node metastasis pelvic and/or para-aortic nodes

Distant Metastasis (M)

MX		Distant metastasis cannot be assessed
M0		No distant metastasis
M1	IVB	Distant metastasis (includes metastasis to abdominal lymph nodes other than para-aortic, and/or inguinal lymph nodes; excludes metastasis to vaginal pelvic serosa, or adnexa)

STAGE GROUPING			
Stage 0	Tis	N0	M0
Stage I	T1	N0	M0
Stage IA	T1a	N0	M0
Stage IB	T1b	N0	M0
Stage IC	T1c	N0	M0
Stage II	T2	N0	M0
Stage IIA	T2a	N0	M0
Stage IIB	T2b	N0	M0

TABLE 8.2. *Continued*

Stage III	T3	N0	M0
Stage IIIA	T3a	N0	M0
Stage IIIB	T3b	N0	M0
Stage IIIC	T1	N1	M0
	T2	N1	M0
	T3	N1	M0
Stage IVA	T4	Any N	M0
Stage IV	Any T	Any N	M1

Source: Used with the permission of the American Joint Committee on Cancer (AJCC), Chicago, Illinois. The original source for this material is the AJCC Cancer Staging Manual, Sixth Edition (2002) published by Springer-New York, www.springeronline.com.

Chapter 9
Normal Uptake and Normal Variant Uptake

The information presented below is a reasonably comprehensive, but not exhaustive, list of common areas of normal and variant uptake seen on FDG-PET/CT scanning. The areas that are illustrated in the images in this chapter are in boldface. In addition, a small number of pathological images are included for comparative purposes.

HEAD AND NECK
Brain gray matter (gray matter more intense than white matter)
Eye muscles (fast twitch muscles with a high glycolytic rate)
Spinal cord
Palatine tonsils
Lingual tonsils (symmetric tonsillar activity)
Adenoids
Vocal cords (patient talking during the uptake phase)
Vocal cords (left recurrent laryngeal nerve palsy)

Prevertebral muscles
Pterygoid muscles
Masseter muscles
Tip of tongue
Ill-fitting dentures
Oral mucosa
Tip of nose
Ears
Sternocleidomastoid muscles
Trapezius muscles
Bifurcation of blood vessels
Blood pool
Brown fat

CHEST

Bifurcation of vessels
Activated plaques
Heart muscle (variable cardiac uptake related to blood glucose level and any areas of ischaemia)
Lung hila
Esophageal uptake
Lactating breast
Nipples
Thymus

ABDOMEN AND PELVIS

Liver
Spleen
Kidneys, ureters, and bladder
Pelvic kidney
Stomach
Pyloric outlet and proximal duodenum
Diffuse, segmental, and focal bowel activity
Cecal pole
Hepatic flexure
Splenic flexure
Low-grade adrenal
Aorta and IVC
Ichial bursitis
Trochanteric bursitis
Bifurcation of vessels
Vaginal reflux
Ovaries
Fibroids
Seminal vesicles
Anal sphincter
Testicular
Perineum

MUSCULOSKELETAL

Any activated muscle
Reactive bone marrow posttherapy or GSF
Healing fractures (e.g., ribs)
Sites of injection (e.g., fragmin, heparin, insulin)
Degenerative or inflammatory joint disease

OTHERS

Inflammation/infection (colonic, lung, vascular)
Granulomatous conditions (e.g., tuberculosis and sarcoidosis)
Thyroid-Thyrotoxicosis

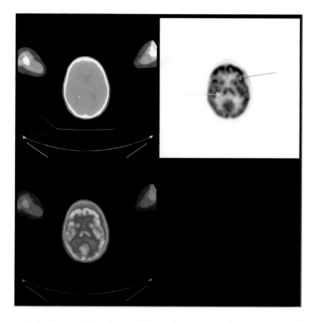

FIGURE 9.1. **Normal brain activity.** This image demonstrates the fact that cortical gray matter has a more intense uptake of FDG than white matter; this reflects the associated glucose metabolism. The gray matter of the basal ganglia can clearly be seen with arrows pointing to the left caudate head (red arrow) and the right thalamus (yellow arrow). The brain uses glucose exclusively as an energy substrate and therefore normal functioning brain cells always have intense FDG uptake associated. Areas of ischemic or infarcted brain are associated with less intense or absent FDG uptake. It is easy to see why the assessment of metastatic lesions to the brain can be difficult using a PET scan. The metastatic deposit would need to have more intense metabolic activity than the normal brain to be identified.

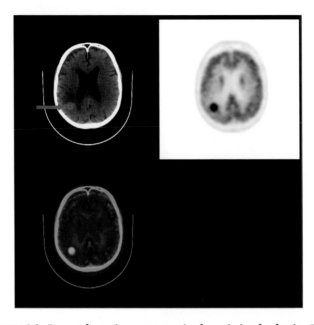

FIGURE 9.2. **Intensely active metastastic deposit in the brain.** This melanoma deposit is identified within the right hemisphere in the posterior parietal cortical gray matter. The corresponding CT image demonstrates a small circular lesion which is of higher attenuation (brighter) than the surrounding brain. This is a common appearance within many melanoma metastases.

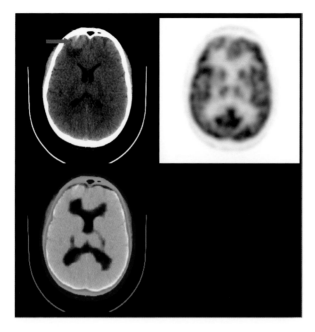

FIGURE 9.3. **An inactive metastatic brain deposit.** This is an image from another patient with disseminated malignant melanoma. On this occasion, the lesion does not have associated FDG uptake, which is an uncommon but documented feature of some melanoma metastases. The high attenuation deposit is identified on the CT component of the study within the cortical gray matter of the right frontal lobe (red arrow).

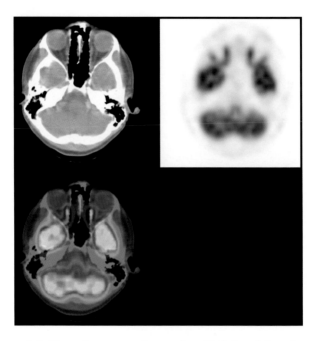

FIGURE 9.4. **Normal eye muscle uptake.** Medial and lateral rectus muscle uptake is commonly found. These muscles are fast twitch muscles and have a high glycolytic rate. The medial recti are usually more intense than the lateral muscles because of their role in accommodation.

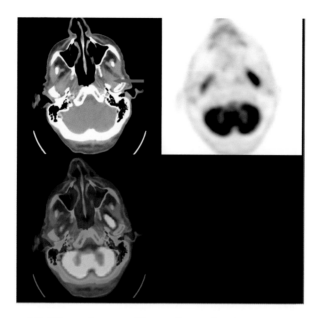

FIGURE 9.5. **Bilateral pterygoid muscle uptake.** Symmetric or asymmetric facial and/or neck muscle uptake is a fairly common occurrence. This is often the result of nervous muscle tension. Several examples are outlined. These patterns are recognizable, and the appearances must be differentiated from pathological processes. FDG uptake within muscles due to tension can often be reduced by the administration of diazepam prior to injection.

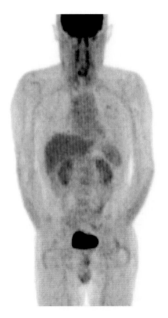

FIGURE 9.6. **MIP view of prevertebral tension-related muscle uptake.**

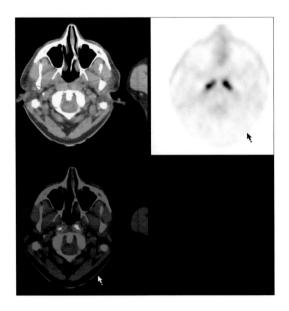

FIGURE 9.7. **Axial view of prevertebral tension-related muscle uptake.**

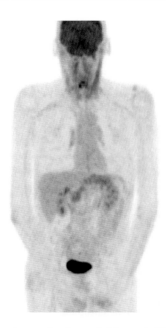

FIGURE 9.8. **MIP view of sternocleidomastoid and low-grade esophageal uptake.** This patient demonstrates physiological uptake within the sternocleidomastoid muscles as well as low-grade FDG uptake in the esophagus. Benign esophageal uptake is a common finding and can cause potential confusion in those patients with suspected gastroesophageal junctional tumors. Tumors of the OG junction can sometimes have extremely low-grade FDG uptake, which could easily be mistaken for physiological uptake of the type seen in this image.

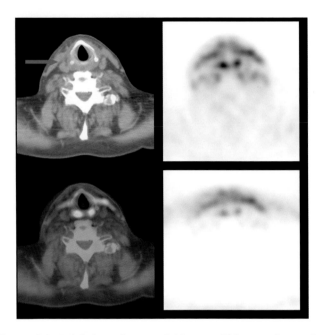

FIGURE 9.9. **Axial view of sternocleidomastoid low-grade uptake.**

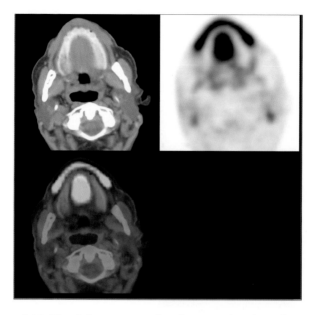

FIGURE 9.10. **Tip of the tongue and oral mucosa.** Uptake in the tongue and oral mucosa are very commonly found and should not be mistaken for pathological processes.

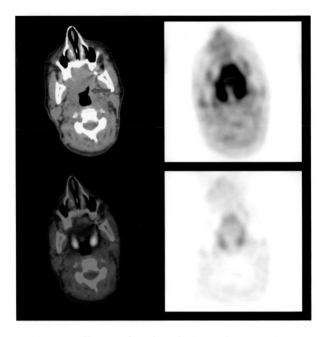

FIGURE 9.11. **Tonsillar uptake.** Physiologic uptake is seen in most individuals. Like other areas of normal uptake in the head and neck, these sites can harbor early malignant change. Careful attention must be paid to minor degrees of asymmetry in cases of head and neck cancer. The left tonsil is indicated by a red arrow.

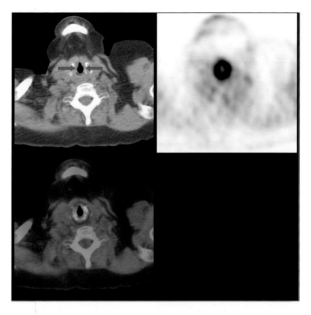

FIGURE 9.12. **Normal vocal cords with symmetric uptake.** This patient talked during the uptake phase of the study.

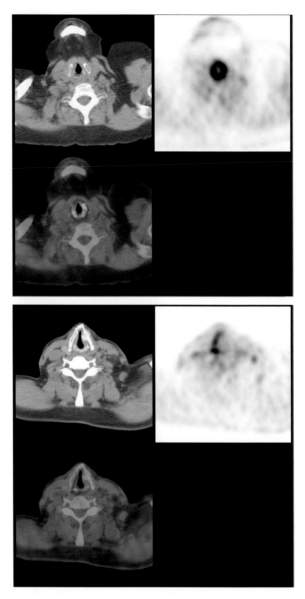

FIGURE 9.13. **Asymmetric vocal cord uptake.** This image shows asymmetric vocal cord uptake with increased uptake in the right cord as compared with the left. Normal vocal cords do not usually show uptake unless the patient has been talking during the uptake period before imaging. In this case, you could be forgiven for thinking that there is abnormal uptake within the right cord. If, however, you were told that the patient has a left hilar lung mass, it becomes clear that the left cord it the abnormal one. The right cord has normal uptake and there is loss of uptake in the left cord due to a left recurrent laryngeal nerve palsy caused by the hilar mass.

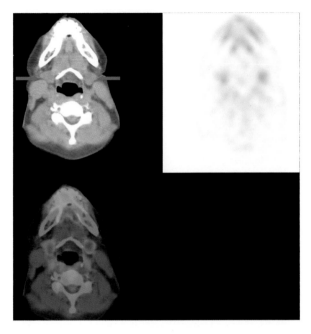

FIGURE 9.14. **Submandibular gland uptake.** Uptake within the salivary glands can be quite variable, but the parotid and submandibular glands are commonly seen.

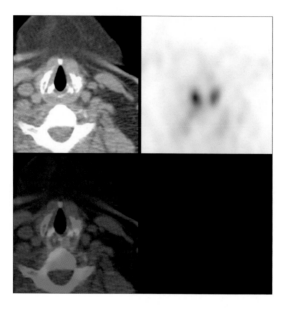

FIGURE 9.15. **Aryetenoid muscle uptake.** The aryetenoid muscles much like the rectus muscles of the eyes are fast twitch muscles and have a high glycolytic rate. These muscles are often seen and, in fact, in this situation uptake acts both as an anatomical landmark on the PET component of the study and as an assessor of patient movement on the fused PET/CT.

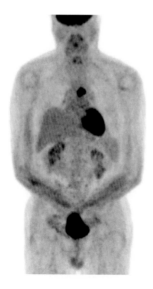

FIGURE 9.16. **MIP view of posttherapy rebound thymic hyperplasia.** The normal thymus is often stunned following the administration of chemotherapeutic agents. In the posttherapy phase, the thymus may become hyperplasic and be identified on the PET/CT scan as an anterior mediastinal soft tissue mass with sometimes intense FDG uptake. In children and young adults, the thymus may be seen as a normal finding on both PET and CT components of the study. The normal thymus involutes in early adult life and is rarely normally demonstrated after the age of 30.

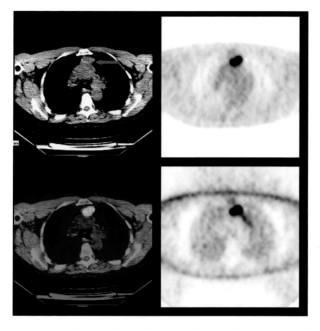

FIGURE 9.17. **Axial view of posttherapy rebound thymic hyperplasia.**

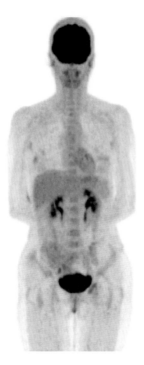

FIGURE 9.18. **Low-grade cardiac uptake.** The uptake of FDG within the heart is extremely variable. Under normal fasting conditions the preferred cardiac energy substrate is actually free fatty acids. Glucose and lipids can also be used if required. If the patient has had a recent glucose meal and a high blood glucose, there will be increased cardiac glucose utilization. This is in part the result of high blood glucose prompting a resultant increase in insulin, which in turn forces glucose into myocardial cells. This is however a very simplistic explanation of the processes involved. Patients with extensive myocardial ischaemic change lose the ability to metabolise free fatty acids efficiently through the normal aerobic pathways. Any such ischemic myocardial cells revert to anaerobic glucose metabolism. In these patients, there will be extensive cardiac glucose metabolism even in a fasting state and as a result there will be marked cardiac FDG uptake seen on the PET scan.

FIGURE 9.19. **Intense cardiac uptake.** The intense cardiac uptake seen in this scan most probably reflects a recent meal. The patient had not followed instructions to fast for four hours prior to the injection of FDG.

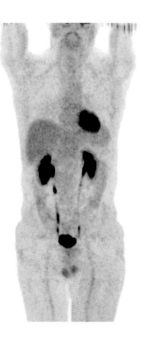

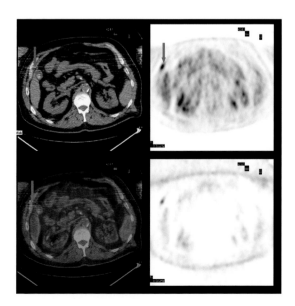

FIGURE 9.20. **Low-grade uptake in a right-sided rib fracture.**

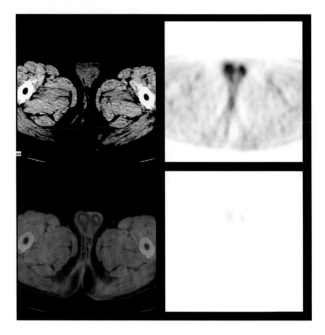

FIGURE 9.21. **Axial view of normal testicular uptake.**

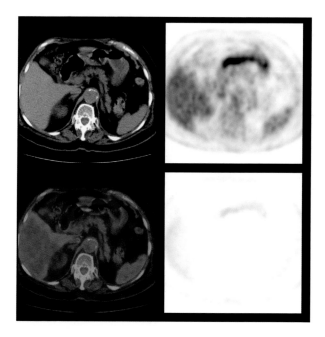

FIGURE 9.22. **FDG uptake within pyloric gastritis.** There are several areas of physiological accumulation of FDG within the bowel. The first and second parts of the duodenum are two such sites. Accumulation of FDG is also commonly found at the distal terminal ileum and caecal pole, where it can simulate active inflammatory bowel disease or even a colonic tumor. Other sites of physiological increased FDG uptake are at the hepatic and splenic flexures, as well as the sigmoid colon and anorectal junction. These sites are all sites of normal physiological hold-up. We must be careful to ensure that FDG uptake at these sites does not actually represent a pathological process and considered evaluation of the CT component of the PET/CT scan is needed.

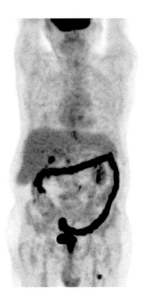

FIGURE 9.23. **Diffuse colonic uptake.** There can be intense diffuse FDG uptake throughout the large (and less commonly the small) bowel. The uptake being related to increased GLUT activity. Attempts have been made to classify increased FDG colonic activity into three recognizable patterns. The first is described as diffuse colonic activity; the second is segmental activity, and the third is focal activity. In general, the diffuse variety rarely relates to any pathological abnormality. Segmental uptake is again most commonly a benign incidental finding, but occasionally it can indicate a segment of inflammatory, infected, or even ischemic bowel. A solitary focal area of colonic FDG uptake is worthy of further evaluation, assuming no obvious abnormality is demonstrated on the CT component of the scan. Sigmoidoscopy or colonoscopy can reveal abnormalities related to the FDG uptake in up to 60% of such cases. Very often the abnormality found relates to an area of mucosal inflammation but early polypoid change has also been detected this way. In approximately 5% of cases an area of frank malignancy will be found.

FIGURE 9.24. **Segmental colonic uptake.** This image reveals segmental uptake along the ascending colon which appeared normal on subsequent colonoscopy. Now review Figure 9.38 and compare how benign and inflammatory uptake can appear very similar.

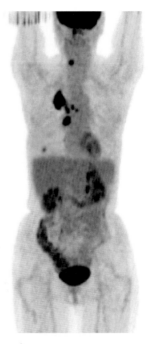

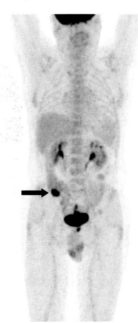

FIGURE 9.25. **Focal colonic uptake.** This focus in the right lower quadrant was due to a adenocarcinoma of the caecum.

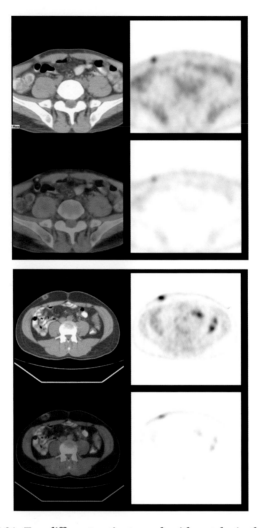

FIGURE 9.26. **Two different patients, each with uptake in the subcu-
taneous fat of the anterior abdominal wall. The focal uptake in each
case in the result of heparin injections.** Injections into the fat overlying the anterior abdominal wall, buttocks or shoulders can appear as
metabolically active soft tissue nodularity.

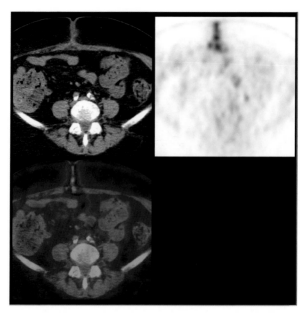

FIGURE 9.27. **Healing midline scar.** There is often metabolic activity within sites of postsurgical change, midline scars, stoma sites, stent insertions, and areas of biopsy or even injection sites. This activity fades with time but for large scars may persist for longer than six months. The appearance is due to metabolically active macrophage accumulation and is caused by a glucose dependant respiratory burst as the macrophage digests tissue debris.

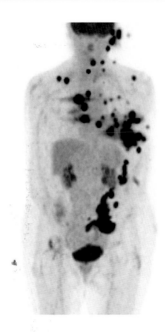

FIGURE 9.28. **Spilled FDG across the patient.** This is an unusual image simulating extensive disease. A closer look reveals that some of the focal sites of FDG uptake lie outside the body. This artefact was due to a leak from the cannula at the site of injection and a subsequent spray of FDG across the patient as her arms were moved above her head.

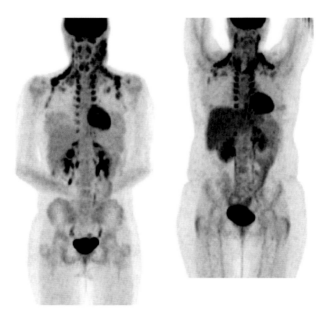

FIGURE 9.29. **Typical patterns of brown fat distribution.** These two different patients demonstrate the typical appearance of diffuse brown fat activation within the neck and thorax. Brown fat is metabolically active fat that has an intense glucose turnover. These same regions can often show **MIBG** (meta-iodo-benzyl-guanidine) uptake in patients injected with this radioactive tracer indicating that brown fat also has a sympathetic nerve innervation. Increased brown fat activation is most commonly found in young thin female patients particularly in cold weather. The activity can be reduced by keeping the patient warm and the use of diazepam which can also help reduce muscle uptake due to nervous tension. If a **PET** scan only had been performed, it would be impossible to confirm that each focal area of **FDG** uptake corresponds to a site of fat and does not represent a soft tissue tumor. The patient on the left has no active disease only activated fat. The patient on the right has activated fat and an active soft tissue mass in the left axilla which represented a lymphomatous recurrence. See Figures 3.19 to 3.21.

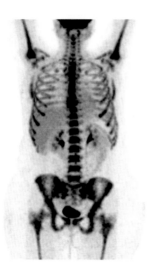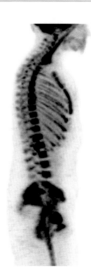

FIGURE 9.30. **Granulocyte-stimulating factor in Hodgkin's disease.** Patients with depleted bone marrow are sometimes given granulocyte-stimulating factor. This has the effect of regenerating marrow production. As a result, the marrow will use considerable amount of glucose to feed marrow proliferation. If a PET/CT scan is performed during this time, the appearances wll reflect the intense marrow activation and an image similar to a bone scan will be obtained. There have been cases of marrow activity so intense that malignant tumors have not been seen. This is because the marrow and any tumor site elsewhere in the body are actively competing for glucose (and thereforeFDG). It is best to wait at least eight weeks after the administration of GSF before carrying out a PET/CT scan.

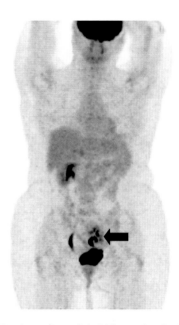

FIGURE 9.31. **MIP view of a pelvic kidney simulating a pathological process.**

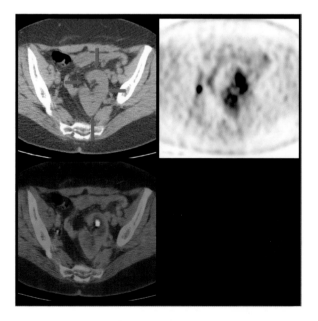

FIGURE 9.32. **Axial view of a pelvic kidney simulating pathological process.**

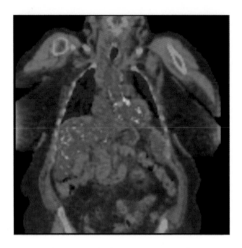

FIGURE 9.33. **Coronal view of abnormal vascular uptake extending along the proximal aortic arch.**

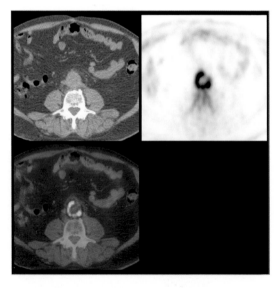

FIGURE 9.34. **Axial view of an area of inflammatory aortitis in the distal thoracic aorta.**

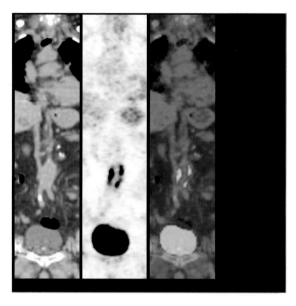

FIGURE 9.35. **Coronal view of inflammatory aortitis of the thoracic aorta.**

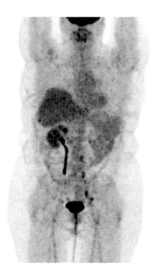

FIGURE 9.36. **Solitary right kidney.**

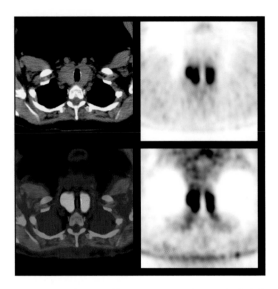

FIGURE 9.37. **Thyroiditis.** Diffuse FDG uptake in both lobes of the thyroid gland in a patient with altered thyroid function tests due to thyroiditis.

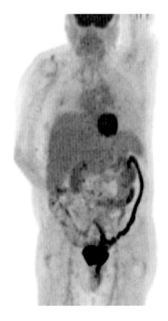

FIGURE 9.38. **Inflammatory bowel disease; this is a confirmed case of ulcerative colitis.**

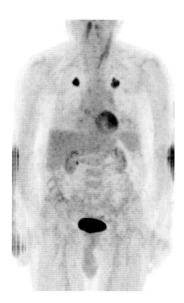

FIGURE 9.39. **Inflammatory lung bilateral sarcoidosis.**

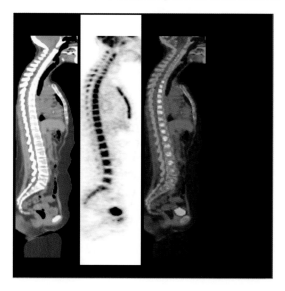

FIGURE 9.40. **Postchemotherapy scan in a patient with a central obstructing left hilar tumor.** Midline sagittal image. As earlier scans have shown, marrow activity need not necessarily represent a maligment process. In this case, the uptake is due to activated regenerating marrow after the insult of earlier chemotherapy.

Chapter 10
Basic Physics

WHAT IS PET?

Positron emission tomography (PET) is a technique that uses radioactive materials known as radionuclides to obtain images that map out metabolic activity in the body. Radionuclides are unstable compounds that decay to more stable compounds by the emission from the nucleus of radioactivity in the form of either particles, photons of energy, or both. The radionuclides commonly used in PET scanning are produced in a device called a cyclotron, and a ring of specialized detectors placed around the patient detects emissions. All radioactive materials decay in an exponential manner with a rate that is characteristic to a specific type of radionuclide.

A cyclotron accelerates a beam of charged particles to very high velocity and then directs this beam into a block of material known as the target. The desired radionuclide can be produced as a result of the changes that take place in the target material due to the bombardment by the high-speed charged particles. The radionuclide produced by the cyclotron can then be attached (labeled) to compounds that are of biological interest, such as glucose, ammonia, or water. The radiolabeled complex is usually injected intravenously and will then distribute throughout the body according to its biological properties.

The most commonly used pairing is the glucose analog 2-deoxy-2-fluoro-D-glucose (FDG) labeled to the radioactive positron emitter fluorine-18. This radiolabeled complex has similar biological properties to glucose and is widely taken up in tissues throughout the body that utilize glucose.

These concepts are outlined in more detail below. A full description of the technology and elemental physics involved in PET/CT is beyond the scope of this book, but see the bibliography if you are adventurous enough to tackle the subject in greater detail.

BASIC NUCLEAR PHYSICS

All matter is comprised of atoms, the smallest possible component into which an element can be broken down without losing its chemical identity. Atoms can be further subdivided into constituent particles. We commonly view the atom as a small compact nucleus consisting of positively charged protons tightly packed close to neutrons, which do not carry any charge. The nucleus is surrounded by a diffuse cloud of orbiting electrons. The electrons are felt to exist in orbits surrounding the nucleus and move without loss of energy. Electrons are extremely small negatively charged particles that weigh less than 1/2000 of either a proton or a neutron. A simple analogy is to imagine the sun as the nucleus of the atom and the planets as the orbiting electrons. Therefore, the majority of an atom is mostly empty space.

In the most stable configuration, the electrons occupy the innermost orbits, where they are most tightly bound by the attraction of the heavy nucleus. Electrons can be moved to higher orbits, but this requires the input of energy to move the electron from the tightly bound orbits to higher orbits. If sufficient energy is delivered to the electron, the atom can be "ionized," that is the electron is completely removed from the atom.

The definition of "radiation" is basically energy in transit. If the energy of the radiation is sufficient to remove an electron from an atom, the radiation is said to be ionizing. Ionizing radiation comes in two main forms. The first form is particulate radiation. This radiation consists of atomic or subatomic particles (alpha particles, protons, electrons, neutrons, positrons, etc) that carry energy in the form of kinetic energy. The second form is electromagnetic radiation (X-rays, Gamma-rays) in which energy is carried by electromagnetic radiation.

> **Top Tip**
> Ionizing radiation has sufficient energy to ionize atoms.

The nucleus of the atom is characterized by both the number of protons and neutrons. The atomic number of the atom is denoted by Z, the number of protons in the nucleus. Each chemical element is defined by a unique number of protons in the nucleus. The mass number of the atom is denoted by A, the total number of protons and neutrons in the nucleus. The common notation for describing nuclear composition is

$$^A_Z X$$

where A is the mass number, Z is the atomic number, and X represents the chemical element to which the atom belongs (e.g., H for Hydrogen ($Z = 1$), He for Helium ($Z = 2$)).

Each chemical element can have a number of different configurations of the nucleus. The number of protons will always remain constant for a given element, but the number of neutrons can differ. Nuclides that have the same atomic number Z but different atomic masses are known as isotopes. For example, hydrogen has three well-known isotopes. All nuclides of hydrogen have one proton. The majority of hydrogen nuclides do not have neutrons in the nucleus. However, hydrogen also comes in isotopes with one neutron (deuteron) and two neutrons (tritium). These three isotopes of hydrogen all behave chemically in the same way, even though the nucleus between the isotopes differs.

Not all combinations of neutrons and protons produce stable nuclides. These unstable nuclides emit energy in the form of particles and/or electromagnetic radiation to transform themselves into a more stable configuration of neutrons and protons. This transformation is the process known as "radioactive decay."

Alpha particles tend to be emitted by heavy elements which need to lose mass to become stable. Alpha particles consist of two protons and two neutrons

$$^A_Z X \xrightarrow{\alpha} {}^{A-4}_{Z-2} Y$$

Electrons (or beta particles, as they are more commonly known when emitted as radiation) tend to be emitted by nuclides with an excess of neutrons. Essentially, a neutron in the nucleus is converted into a proton and an electron. The proton is retained within the nucleus and the electron is emitted with kinetic energy.

$$^A_Z X \xrightarrow{\beta-} {}^{A}_{Z+1} Y$$

DECAY AND DETECTION OF POSITRONS
Positron Physics
What is a positron? Basically, a positron is an antielectron or, in other words, a positively charged electron. Antimatter does actually exist and is not just a figment of Captain Kirk's imagination. All particles mentioned in this chapter have an antimatter version (e.g., antiproton). Without going into the complexities of what antimatter actually is, the positron can be though of as an

electron with a positive charge. Positrons are produced by nuclei that are unstable and have an excess of protons.

$$\prescript{A}{Z}{X} \xrightarrow{\beta+} \prescript{A}{Z-1}{Y}$$

When an atom undergoes radioactive decay by positron emission, a proton in the nucleus is transformed into a neutron and a positron. The positron is then ejected from the nucleus with a very small uncharged mass called a neutrino carrying off a variable amount of excess energy.

The positron is highly unstable outside the nucleus and seeks to combine with a nearby electron to from a positronium ion. This ion is also unstable and disintegrates (annihilates) by the conversion of its mass into pure energy. This process is governed by Einstein's mass-energy principle, which states that a particle of mass M can be converted into energy E by the equation $E = Mc^2$, where c is the speed of light. Since the mass of the positronium ion is known we are able to calculate the amount of energy that will be obtained, 1022 KeV. This energy is in the form of two photons, which share the total energy equally, 511 KeV each and are emitted simultaneously in opposite directions following annihilation (Figure 10.1).

The annihilation process takes place extremely rapidly (within 2 nanoseconds) following the emission of the positron from the nucleus, in general occurring no more than 1 mm to

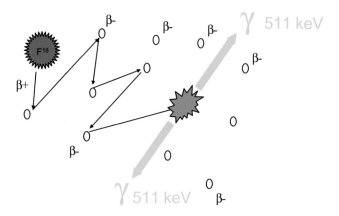

FIGURE 10.1. Positron interactions.

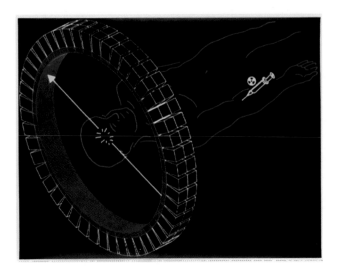

FIGURE 10.2. 411 keV coincidence detection.

2 mm from the atom that emitted the positron. The basic physics on which PET imaging is based is the detection of these two simultaneous opposing gamma ray photons generated by every decay event.

A ring of detectors (Figure 10.2) surrounds the patient and can accurately detect the photons emitted as a result of the annihilation process. Since the annihilation occurs about two millimeters from the decaying nucleus, we can therefore demonstrate accurately the site of FDG uptake in the body.

Top Tip
It is not the short-lived positrons that are detected in our positron emission tomography scanners, but in fact gamma ray photons that are emitted as a result of the annihilation of the positron.

Production of PET Radiotracers
For a nucleus to emit positrons, it must be unstable and have a surplus of protons. Therefore to manufacture positron-emitting radionuclides, a method must be used to add protons into stable

nuclei. This is achieved in a device called a cyclotron. The cyclotron has a source of charged particles that are accelerated using a magnetic field to very high energies, creating enough energy to penetrate the nucleus of a suitable target material. For example, to produce the positron-emitting fluoride-18 ion, a target of oxygen-18 enriched water is bombarded in a cyclotron by a beam of high-energy protons.

Cyclotrons

The majority of positron emitting radioisotopes used in PET are produced in cyclotrons, although high energy linear accelerators have occasionally been used. The first cyclotron was built in 1930 and the basic principle involves the acceleration of charged particles (protons, deuterons, $^3H^{++}$, and α particles) in a circular path by the application of radiofrequency and magnetic field but without the use of high voltages (see Figure 10.3.)

Particle acceleration takes place inside hollow metal cavities known as Dees (A and B). The dees are connected to a radiofrequency oscillator to supply potential so that their polarities can be alternated. The ion source S is placed in the center of the gap between the two dees. Ions are normally produced by the ionization of an appropriate gas using an electrical arc (e.g., protons from ionization if H_2 gas).

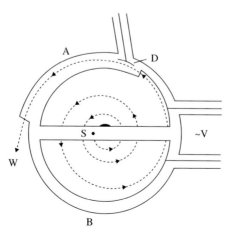

FIGURE 10.3. Schematic of a cyclotron.

A positive particle will be accelerated toward the negative dee. Once inside the dee, the particle will no longer be under the influence of the electrical field, but a magnetic field perpendicular to the place of the dee will force it to move in a circular path. When the particle again reaches the gap, the polarity of the dees is changed and the particle is accelerated towards the other dee. The velocity of the particle has increased, so it will traverse a path with a larger radius within the dee. The radiofrequency oscillators are tuned such that the change in polarities is in phase with the arrival of the particles in the gap. Each time the charged particle crosses the gap it gains kinetic energy. As the ions reach the periphery of the dees, the beam of particles is removed by an oppositely charged deflector plate and allowed through a window to be used for the irradiation of targets.

The targets are designed for the production of specific radionuclides such as carbon 11, nitrogen 13, oxygen 15, and fluorine 18, the most commonly used radionuclides in PET. When the target is hit by the charged particle beam, the charged particle deposits its energy into the nucleus of the target nucleus. The target nucleus then emits proton and neutrons until all of the excitation energy is disposed of, producing a different radionuclide. The yield of each radionuclide depends upon the beam intensity, amount of target material bombarded, the cross section for the production of the radionucilde and time of bombardment.

The radioisotopes are passed through automated black boxes which synthesize the common PET radiopharmaceuticals. The boxes contain hardware such as glassware, tubing, pipetting mechanism and the necessary chemicals and are computer controlled.

^{11}C, ^{13}N, and ^{15}O are of great interest, as they are constituents in all biologic substances. One of the characteristics of radioactive materials is half-life. The half-life is specific to each radionuclide. In general, PET radionuclides have a very short half-life. Fluorine 18 has a half life of 110 minutes. This means that it is possible to create the fluorine 18, manufacture the radiopharmaceutical, transport the radiopharmaceutical to a distant site, and still have enough activity to perform a scan.

Unfortunately, the half lives of ^{11}C, ^{13}N, and ^{15}O are much shorter than ^{18}F. This means that they can only be used on a site with a dedicated biomedical cyclotron. The high cost of owning such a machine has prevented their widespread use. However, in the past ten years, there has been a significant increase in the use of PET thoughout the world, and the number of cyclotrons in hospital locations has mushroomed.

After cyclotron production, the positron-emitting radio-nuclides have to be incorporated into radiopharmaceuticals that can be administered into the human body. This is achieved by a process of radiolabeling in a specialized radiochemistry facility. For example, the fluoride-18 ion is incorporated into 2-deoxy-2-fluoro-D-glucose to form ^{18}FDG. PET radionuclides are also easily incorporated into biochemically relevant molecules because of their small size.

Generator Produced Positron Emitting Radionuclides

Not all radioisotopes that emit positrons have to be produced in a cyclotron. There are several generator produced positron emitting radioisotopes that have been used clinically. These include positron emitting radionuclides of rubidium, copper, and gallium.

PET Scanner Design

The PET scanner is designed to detect simultaneously the oppos-ing 511 keV gamma rays produced during the positron-electron annihilation events. Most PET scanners are made up of a series of bismuth germinate (BGO) scintillation detectors configured in rings around the patient. Up to 20,000 detector crystals may be used in one scanner covering a length of about 15 cm of the patient's body at any time. Detector crystals are grouped together in detector blocks and are connected to photomultiplier tubes and other electronic circuitry that detect the gamma ray emis-sions and convert them into electrical signals. The electrical signals are used to determine the location of the positron-electron annihilation events. To complete a whole-body PET scan, the scanning bed (and patient) must be moved every few minutes so that each part of the body is consecutively within the detector rings.

Every time a photon pair is detected simultaneously, the system assumes that these have come from the same annihila-tion interaction and creates one event lying on the line joining the two detectors. Millions of these lines are acquired and merged to form a picture of where the annihilation event occurred, which is therefore very close to the position from which the positron was emitted. By reviewing all the detector pairs and lines of responses, a three-dimensional distribution of the radiotracer can be reconstructed. The method of iterative reconstruction is most commonly used to rebuild the picture of the radiotracer distribution in the body.

WHAT IS PET/CT?

Unfortunately the resolution of the PET system is not sufficient to provide the accurate anatomical localization of a CT scanner. The CT scanner of course can only provide anatomical information but no indication of metabolic activity. Technology has now advanced sufficiently to apply these two modalities almost simultaneously to produce an image. This fusion image combines the CT anatomical data with the metabolic uptake identified by the PET component. This allows us to accurately map out the anatomical distribution of metabolic function.

Following the intravenous injection of the radioactive tracer, uptake continues in metabolically active tissues for some time. Most centers allow uptake to continue for 45 minutes to 1 hour before imaging takes place. During this uptake period, the patient is asked to lie still in a darkened room to prevent unnecessary movement or stimulation. Any muscle movement or talking during the uptake phase will result in physiological uptake, which will be later visible on the scan.

The CT scan is acquired first with the patient lying supine in a relaxed pose with arms folded across their abdomen. Nowadays a 16 or 32 slice CT scanner can perform a whole body scan in only a few seconds. The normal range is from the base of skull to upper thighs only. The brain is not routinely included, as the marked FDG uptake from the normal brain makes detection of metabolically active lesions difficult (but not impossible). In certain circumstances, the range may be extended to include the head and neck. An example would be if the patient has known lymphomatous involvement of the cervical nodes or brain. Whole body images are mandatory when scanning patients with melanoma, as the drainage pattern of metastatic disease is so unpredictable.

After the CT scan the patient is asked to remain in the same position (with head restraints used if head and neck images are needed). The PET images are then acquired. Each image is acquired for 3 to 5 minutes over a range of about 15 centimeters in the craniocaudal direction, meaning that the whole range, from skull base to upper thighs, takes about 45 minutes.

The Problem of Attenuation

As gamma rays pass through the body, they lose some of their energy. This is known as attenuation. Different tissues reduce the energy of the gamma rays by different amounts because of their various densities. To build up an accurate picture of the 3D distribution of radioactivity within the body, the attenuation of the various tissues and organs must be taken into account. This is best achieved by measuring accurate attenuation data by transmitting a known beam of radiation through the body and measuring its output. Knowing the input and output values of the beam allows us to calculate the degree of attenuation caused by the body. Different body parts will attenuate the beam by different amounts. For example the air-filled lungs will attenuate radiation much less than the soft tissue viscera of the pelvis and its surrounding bony pelvis. This process can sometimes lead to artefacts due to rapid changes in attenuation values around metallic foreign bodies, such as pacemakers, metallic dental work, and hip replacements. Artefacts can also occur due to respiratory motion near the diaphragm, and the use of either oral and in particular intravenous contrast media.

In a PET/CT scanner attenuation, correction maps are created from the CT scanner anatomical images. This allows a more accurate representation of the true distribution of metabolic activity within the body. If artefacts do occur, they usually manifest as areas of increased activity known as hotspots. They are the result of overcorrection of the PET images due to metallic density. In these cases, the nonattenuated PET image should be reviewed to distinguish between abnormal increased activity and technical overcorrection artefact. Real pathology should still persist on the nonattenuated image, whereas the artefact should not.

Attenuation is not the only problem requiring correction in the PET scanner. Not all events detected by the scanner are "true" annihilation events. Some are "random" coincidences, and some are detected from "scattered" events. Random coincidence events occur when two photons arising from different positron decays hit the detector ring at the same time. Scattered coincidences occur when one of the photons is deflected by an atom within the patient and its direction is altered slightly. These are detected by the system as if they were true events. These may lead to a "blurring" of the true position of the event. PET scanners have various in-built methods for trying to correct for some of these errors.

Computer reconstruction is most often carried out using a process known as iterative reconstruction. When this is complete the images are ready to be viewed and can be displayed as CT only, PET only, or a combined PET/CT fused image.

PET/CT is widely felt to provide a significant advantage over PET imaging alone. It allows for precise anatomical location of areas of abnormal metabolic uptake leading to an increased diagnostic accuracy when compared with viewing PET alone or even PET and CT side by side.

Bibliography

CHAPTER I

Beuthien-Baumann B, Hamacher K, Oberdorfer F, Steinbach J. Preparation of fluorine-18 labeled sugars and derivatives and their application as tracer for positron emission-tomography. *Carbohydr Res* 2000; 327:107–118.

Beyer T, Townsend DW, Brun T, et al. A combined PET/CT scanner for clinical oncology. *J Nucl Med* 2000;41:1369–1379.

Cook GJ, Fogelman I, Maisey MN. Normal physiological and benign pathological variants of 18-fluoro-2-deoxyglucose positron-emission tomography scanning: potential for error in interpretation. *Semin Nucl Med* 1996;26(4):308–314.

Cook GJ, Maisey MN, Fogelman I. Normal variants, artefacts and interpretative pitfalls in PET imaging with 18-flouro-2-deoxyglucose and carbon-11 methionine. *Eur J Nucl Med* 1999;26(10):1363–1378.

Fowler JS, Ido T. Initial and subsequent approach for the synthesis of 18FDG. *Semin Nucl Med* 2002;32:6–12.

Gordon BA, Flanagan FL, Dehdashti F. Whole body positron emission tomography: normal variations, pitfalls and technical considerations. *AJR Am J Roentgenol* 1997;169(6):1675–1680.

Gorospe L, Raman S, Echeveste J, et al. Spectrum of physiological variants, artefacts, and interpretative pitfalls in cancer patients. *Nucl Med Commum* 2005;26(8):671–687.

Hoffman EJ, Phelps ME. *Positron emission tomography: principles and quantitation*. New York: Raven Press;1986: pp 237–286.

Keyes JW Jr. SUV: standard uptake or silly useless value? *J Nucl Med* 1995;36:1836–1839.

Cherry SR, Sorenson JA, Phelps ME. *Physics in Nuclear Medicine*, 3rd ed. Philadelphia: Saunders; 2003.

Shreve PD, Anzai Y, Wahl RL. Pitfalls in oncological diagnosis with FDG PET imaging: physiological and benign variants. *Radiographics* 1999; 19(1):61–77.

Thie JA. Understanding the standardized uptake value, its methods, and implications for usage. *J Nucl Med* 2004;45:1431–1434.

Warburg O, et al. The metabolism of cancer cells. *Biochem Zeitschr* 1924;152:129–169.

Zasadny KR, Wahl RL. Standardized uptake values of normal tissues with FDG: variation with body weight and method for correction. *Radiology* 1993;189(3):847–850.

CHAPTER 2

Ahuja V, Coleman RE, Herndon J, et al. The prognostic significance of fluorodeoxyglucose positron emission tomography imaging for patients with nonsmall cell lung carcinoma. *Cancer* 1998;83:918–924.

Arita T, Kuramitsu T, Kawamura M. Bronchogenic carcinoma: incidence of metastases to normal sized lymph nodes. *Thorax* 1995;50:1267–1269.

Bradley JD, Dehdashti F, Mintun MA, Govindan R, Trinkaus K, Siegel BA. Positron emission tomography in limited-stage small-cell lung cancer: a prospective study. *J Clin Oncol* 2004;22:3248.

Brink I, Schumacher T, Mix M, et al. Impact of [18F]FDG-PET on the primary staging of small-cell lung cancer. *Eur J Nucl Med Mol Imaging* 2004;31:1614–1620.

Cerfolio RJ, Ojha B, Bryant AS, Raghuveer V, Mountz JM, Bartolucci AA. The accuracy of integrated PET-CT compared with dedicated PET alone for the staging of patients with non-small cell lung cancer. *Ann Thorac Surg* 2004;78:1017–1023.

Detterbeck FC, Falen S, Rivera MP, Halle JS, Socinski MA. Seeking a home for a PET, I: defining the appropriate place for positron emission tomography imaging in the diagnosis of pulmonary nodules or masses. *Chest* 2004;125:2294–2299.

Detterbeck FC, Vansteenkiste JF, Morris DE, Dooms CA, Khandani AH, Socinski MA. Seeking a home for a PET, III: emerging applications of positron emission tomography imaging in the management of patients with lung cancer. *Chest* 2004;126:1656–1666.

Dhital K, Saunders CA, Seed PT, et al. [18F]Fluorodeoxyglucose positron emission tomography and its prognostic value in lung cancer. *Eur J Cardiothorac Surg* 2000;18:425–428.

Gambhir SS, Shepherd JE, Shah BD, et al. Analytical decision model for the cost-effective management of solitary pulmonary nodules. *J Clin Oncol* 1998;16:2113–2125.

Gould MK, Maclean CC, Kuschner WG, Rydzak CE, Owens DK. Accuracy of positron emission tomography for diagnosis of pulmonary nodules and mass lesions: a meta-analysis. *JAMA* 2001;285:914–924.

Greene FL, Page DL, Fleming ID, et al. *AJCC Cancer Staging Manual*, Sixth Edition. New York: Springer, 2002.

Hauber HP, Bohuslavizki KH, Lund CH, et al. PET in the staging of small cell lung cancer. *Chest* 2001;119:950–954.

Herder GJ, Golding RP, Hoekstra OS, et al. The performance of (18)F-fluorodeoxyglucose positron emission tomography in small solitary pulmonary nodules. *Eur J Nucl Med Mol Imaging* 2004;31:1231–1236.

Higashi K, Ueda Y, Arisaka Y, et al. FDG uptake as a biologic prognostic factor for recurrence in patients with surgically resected non-small cell lung cancer. *J Nucl Med* 2002;43:39–45.

Jeong HJ, Min JJ, Park JM, et al. Determination of the prognostic value of [(18)F]fluorodeoxyglucose uptake by using positron emission tomography in patients with non-small cell lung cancer. *Nucl Med Commun* 2002;23:865–870.

Lardinois D, Weder W, Hany TF, et al. Staging of non-small-cell lung cancer with integrated positron-emission tomography and computed tomography. *N Engl J Med* 2003;348:2500–2507.

MacManus, MP, Hicks RJ, Matthews JP, et al. Positron emission tomography is superior to computed tomography scanning for response-assessment after radical radiotherapy or chemoradiotherapy in patients with non-small-cell lung cancer. *J Clin Oncol* 2003;21:1285–1292.

Midthun DE. Solitary pulmonary nodule. *Curr Opin Pulm Med* 2000;6:364–370.

Nestle U, Walter K, Schmidt S, et al. FDG PET for the planning of radiotherapy in lung cancer: high impact in patients with atelectasis. *Int J Radiat Oncol Biol Phys* 1999;44:593–597.

Nomori H, Watanabe K, Ohtsuka T, Naruke T, Suemasu K, Uno K. Evaluation of F-18 fluorodeoxyglucose (FDG) PET scanning for pulmonary nodules less than 3 cm in diameter, with special reference to the CT images. *Lung Cancer* 2004;45:19–27.

Pieterman R, van PuttenJ, Meuzelaar J, et al. Preoperative staging of non-small cell lung cancer with PET. *N Engl J Med* 2000;343:254–261.

Port JL, Kent MS, Korst RJ, et al. Positron emission tomography scanning poorly predicts response to preoperative chemotherapy in non-small cell lung cancer. *Ann Thorac Surg* 2004;77:254–259.

Reed CE, Harpole DH, Posther KE, et al. Results of the American College of Surgeons Oncology Group Z0050 trial: the utility of positron emission tomography in staging potentially operable non-small cell lung cancer. *J Thorac Cardiovasc Surg* 2003;126:1943–1951.

Rohren EM, Lowe VJ. Update in PET imaging of non-small cell lung cancer. *Semin Nucl Med* 2004;34:134–153.

Shon IH, O'Doherty MJ, Maisey NM: Positron emission tomography in lung cancer. *Sem Nucl Med* 2002;32:240–271.

Vansteenkiste JF, Stroobants SG. Positron emission tomography in the management of non-small cell lung cancer. *Hematol Oncol Clin North Am* 2004;18:269–288.

van Tinteren H. Hoekstra OS, Smit EF, et al. Effectiveness of positron emission tomography in the preoperative assessment of patients with suspected non-small-cell lung cancer: the PLUS multicentre randomized trial. *Lancet* 2002;359:1388–1393.

Weber, WA, Petersen, V, Schmidt, B, et al. Positron emission tomography in non-small-cell lung cancer: prediction of response to chemotherapy by quantitative assessment of glucose use. *J Clin Oncol* 2003;21,2651–2657.

CHAPTER 3

Allen-Auerbach M, Quon A, Weber WA, et al. Comparison between 2-deoxy-2-[18F]fluoro-D-glucose positron emission tomography and positron emission tomography/computed tomography hardware fusion for staging of patients with lymphoma. *Mol imaging Biol* 2004;6: 411–416.

Barrington SF, O'Doherty MJ. Limitations of PET for imaging lymphoma. *Eur J Nucl Med Mol Imaging* 2003;30:S117–127.

Buchmann I, Reinhardt M, Elsner K, et al. FDG PET in the detection and staging of malignant lymphoma. *Cancer* 2001;91:889–89914.

Depas G, De Barsy C, Jerusalem G, et al. 18F-FDG PET in children with lymphomas. *Eur J Nucl Med Mol Imaging* 2005;32:31–38.

Elstrom R, Guan L, Baker G, et al. Utility of FDG-PET scanning in lymphoma by WHO classification. *Blood* 2003;101:3875–3876.

Filmont JE, Czerin J, Yap C, et al. Value of FDG-PET for predicting the clinical outcome of patients with aggressive lymphoma prior to and after stem cell transplantation. *Chest* Aug 2003;124(2):608–613.

Hermann S, Wormanns D, Pixberg M et al. Staging in childhood lymphoma: differences between FDG-PET and CT. *Nuklearmedizin* 2005; 44:1–7.

Israel O, Keidar Z, Bar-Shalom R. Positron emission tomography in the evaluation of lymphoma. *Semin Nucl Med* 2004;34:166–179.

Jerusalem G, Beguin Y, Fassotte MF, et al. Early detection of relapse by PET in the follow up of patients with Hodgkin's disease. *Ann Oncol* Jan 2003;14(1):123–130.

Jerusalem G, Beguin Y, Fasotte M, et al. Whole body PET using FDG for post treatment evaluation in HD and NHL. *Blood* 1999;94:429–433.

Jerusalem G, Beguin Y, Najjar F, et al. Positron emission tomography (PET) with 18F-fluorodeoxyglucose (18F-FDG) for the staging of low-grade non-Hodgkin's lymphoma (NHL). *Ann Oncol* 2001;12:825–830.

Juweid ME, Wiseman GA, Vose JM, et al. Response assessment of aggressive NHL. *J Clin Oncol* 2005;23:4652–4661.

Klose T, Leidl R, Buchmann I, Brambs HJ, Reske SN. Primary staging of lymphomas: cost-effectiveness of FDG-PET versus computed tomography. *Eur J Nucl Med* 2000;27:1457–1464.

Kostakoglu L, Goldsmith SJ. 18F-FDG PET evaluation of the response to therapy for lymphoma and for breast, lung and colorectal carcinoma. *J Nucl Med* 2003;44:224–239.

Mikhaeel NG, Hutchings M, Fields PA, et al. FDG-PET after two to three cycles of chemotherapy predicts progression-free and overall survival in high-grade non-Hodgkin lymphoma. *Ann Oncol* 2005;16:1514–1523.

Reske SN. PET and restaging of malignant lymphoma including residual masses and relapse. *Eur J Nucl Med Mol Imaging* 2003;30(Suppl 1): S89–S96.

Rini JN, Manalili EY, Hoffman MA, et al. F-18 FDG versus Ga-67 for detecting splenic involvement in Hodgkin's disease. *Clin Nucl Med* 2002;27:572–577.

Sasaki M, Yuwabara Y, Koga H, et al. Clinical impact of whole body FDG PET on staging malignant lymphoma. *Ann Nuc Med* 2002;16:337–345.

Schiepers C, Filmont JE, Czernin J. PET for staging of Hodgkin's disease and non-Hodgkin's lymphoma. *Eur J Nucl Med Mol Imaging* 2003; 30(Suppl 1):S82–S88.

Spaepen K, Stoobants S, Dupont P, et al. Prognostic value of PET with FDG after first line chemotherapy in NHL. *J Clin Oncol* 2001;19: 414–419.

Spaepen K, Stroobants S, Verhoef G, Mortelmans L. Positron emission tomography with [(18)F]FDG for therapy response monitoring in lymphoma patients. *Eur J Nucl Med Mol Imaging* 2003;30(Suppl 1): S97–105.

Stumpe K, Urbinelli M, Steinert H, et al. Whole body positron emission tomography using FDG for staging of lymphoma: effectiveness and comparison with CT. *Eur J Nucl Med* 1998;206:475–481.

Torizuka T, Nakmura F, Kanno T, et al. Early therapy monitoring with FDG PET in aggressive NHL and HD. *Eur J Nucl Med Mol Imaging* 2004;31(1):22–28.

Wegner EA, Barrington SF, Kingston JE et al. The impact of PET scanning on management of paediatric oncology patients. *Eur J Nucl Med Mol Imaging* 2005;32:23–30.

Zinzani PL, Fanti S, Battista G, et al. Predictive role of PET in the outcome of Lymphoma patients. *Br J Cancer* 2004;31,91(5):850–854.

CHAPTER 4

Arslan N, Miller TR, Dehdashti F, et al. Evaluation of response to neoadjuvant therapy by quantitative FDG PET in patients with esophageal cancer. *Mol Imaging Biol* 2002;4:301–310.

Blot W, Devesa S, Kneller R, Fraumeni R. Rising incidence of adenocarcinoma of the esophagus and gastric cardia. *JAMA* 1991;265:1287–1289.

Brucher BL, Weber W, Bauer M, et al. Neoadjuvant therapy of esophageal squamous cell carcinoma: response evaluation by positron emission tomography. *Ann Surg* 2001;233:300–309.

Choi JY, Jang HJ, Shim YM, et al. 18F-FDG PET in patients with esophageal squamous cell carcinoma undergoing curative surgery: prognostic implications. *J Nucl Med* 2004;45:1843–1850.

Downey RJ, Akhurst T, Ilson D, et al. Whole body 18FDG-PET and the response of esophageal cancer to induction therapy: results of a prospective trial. *J Clin Oncol* 2003;21:428–432.

Flamen P, Lerut A, Van CE, et al. Utility of positron emission tomography for the diagnosis and staging of recurrent esophageal cancer. *J Thorac Cardiovasc Surg* 2000;120:1085–1092.

Flamen P, Lerut A, Van CE, et al. Utility of positron emission tomography for the staging of patients with potentially operable esophageal carcinoma. *J Clin Oncol* 2000;18:3202–3210.

Greene FL, Page DL, Fleming ID, et al. *AJCC Cancer Staging Manual*, Sixth Edition. New York: Springer, 2002.

Himeno S, Yasuda S, Shimada H, Tajima T, Makuuchi H. Evaluation of esophageal cancer by positron emission tomography. *Jpn J Clin Oncol* 2002;32:340–346.

Kato H, Miyazaki T, Nakajima M, et al. The incremental effect of positron emission tomography on diagnostic accuracy in the initial staging of esophageal carcinoma. *Cancer* 2005;103:148–156.

Kole A, Plukke RJ, Nieweg O, Vaalburg W. Positron emission tomography for staging of esophageal and gastric malignancy. *Br J Cancer* 1998;78: 521–527.

Lerut T, Flamen P, Ectors N, et al. Histopathologic validation of lymph node staging with FDG-PET scan in cancer of the esophagus and gastroesophageal junction: a prospective study based on primary surgery with extensive lymphadenectomy. *Ann Surg* 2000;232:743–752.

Lightdale C. Staging of esophageal cancer. Endoscopic ultrasonography. *Semin Oncol* 1994;21:438–446.

Luketich JD, Friedman DM, Weigel TL, et al. Evaluation of distant metastases in esophageal cancer: 100 consecutive positron emission tomography scans. *Ann Thorac Surg* 1999;68:1133–1136.

Ott K, Fink U, Becker K, et al. Prediction of response to preoperative chemotherapy in gastric carcinoma by metabolic imaging: results of a prospective trial. *J Clin Oncol* 2003;21:4604–4610.

Swisher SG, Maish M, Erasmus JJ, et al. Utility of PET, CT, and EUS to identify pathologic responders in esophageal cancer. *Ann Thorac Surg* 2004;78:1152–1160.

van Westreenen HL, Westerterp M, Bossuyt PM, et al. Systematic review of the staging performance of 18F-flurodeoxyglucose positron emission tomography in esophageal cancer. *J Clin Oncol* 2004;22:3805–3812.

Wallace MB, Nietert PJ, Earle C, et al. An analysis of multiple staging management strategies for carcinoma of the esophagus: computed tomography, endoscopic ultrasound, positron emission tomography, and thoracoscopy/laparoscopy. *Ann Thorac Surg* 2002;74:1026–1032.

Weber WA, Ott K, Becker K, et al. Prediction of response to preoperative chemotherapy in adenocarcinoma of the esophagogastric junction by metabolic imaging. *J Clin Oncol* 2001;19:3058–3065.

Wieder HA, Brucher BL, Zimmermann F, et al. Time course of tumor metabolic activity during chemoradiotherapy of esophageal squamous cell carcinoma and response to treatment. *J Clin Oncol* 2004;22,900–908.

Yoon YC, Lee KS, Shim YM, et al. Metastasis to regional lymph nodes in patients with esophageal squamous cell carcinoma: CT versus FDG PET for presurgical detection a prospective study. *Radiology* 2003;227: 764–770.

Yoshioka T, Yamaguchi K, Kubota K, et al. Evaluation of 18F-FDG PET in patients with a, metastatic, or recurrent gastric cancer. *J Nucl Med* 2003;44:690–699.

CHAPTER 5

Delbeke D, Vitola J, Sandler MP, et al. Staging recurrent colorectal carcinoma with PET. *J Nucl Med* 1997;38:1196–1201.

Donckier V, Van Laethem JL, Goldman S, et al. FDG-PET as a tool for early recognition of incomplete tumor destruction after radiofrequency ablation for liver metastases. *J Surg Oncol* 2003;84:215–223.

Drenth JP, Nagengast FM, Oyen WJ. Evaluation of premalignant colonic abnormalities: endoscopic validation of FDG-PET findings. *Eur J Nucl Med* 2001;28:1766–1769.

Even-Sapir E, Parag Y, Lerman H, et al. Detection of recurrence in patients with rectal cancer: PET/CT after abdominoperineal or anterior resection. *Radiology* 2004;232:815–822.

Fernandez FG, Drebin JA, Linehan DC, Dehdashti F, Siegel BA, Strasberg SM. Five-year survival after resection of hepatic metastases from colorectal cancer in patients screened by positron emission tomography with F-18 fluorodeoxyglucose (FDG-PET). *Ann Surg* 2004;240:438–447.

Flanagan FL, Dehdashti F, Ogunbiyi OA, et al. Utility of FDG-PET for investigating unexplained plasma CEA evaluation in patients with colorectal cancer. *Ann Surg* 1998;227:319–323.

Fong Y, Saldinger P, Akhurst T, et al. Utility of 18F-FDG positron emission tomography scanning on selection of patients for resection of hepatic colorectal metastases. *Am J Surg*1999;178:282–287.

Greene FL, Page DL, Fleming ID, et al. *AJCC Cancer Staging Manual*, Sixth Edition. New York: Springer, 2002.

Heriot AG, Hicks RJ, Drummond EG, et al. Does positron emission tomography change management in primary rectal cancer? A prospective assessment. *Dis Colon Rectum* 2004;47:451–458.

Heubner RH, Park KC, Sheperd JE, et al. A meta-analysis of the literature for whole body FDG PET detection of recurrent colorectal cancer. *J Nucl Med* 2000;41:1177–1189.

Kostakoglu L, Goldsmith SJ. 18F-FDG PET evaluation of the response to therapy for lymphoma and for breast, lung and colorectal carcinoma. *J Nucl Med* 2003;44:224–239.

Lai DT, Fulham M, Stephen MS, et al. The role of whole body positron emission tomography with FDG in identifying operable colorectal cancer metastases to the liver. *Arch Surg* 1996;131:703–707.

Meyer M. Diffusely increased colonic F-18 FDG uptake in acute enterocolitis. *Clin Nucl Med.* 1995;20:434–435.

Schiepers C, Penninckx F, De Vadder N, et al. Contribution of PET in the diagnosis of recurrent colorectal cancer: comparison with conventional imaging. *Eur J Surg Oncol.* 1995;21:517–522.

Selzner M, Hany TF, Wildbrett P, McCormack L, Kadry Z, Clavien PA. Does the novel PET/CT imaging modality impact on the treatment of patients with metastatic colorectal cancer of the liver? *Ann Surg* 2004; 240:1027–1034.

Tatlidil R, Jadvar H, Bading JR, Conti PS. Incidental colonic FDG uptake: correlation with colonoscopy and histopathology. *Radiology* 2002;224: 783–787.

CHAPTER 6

Adam S, Baum R, Stuckensen T, Bitter K, Hor G. Prospective comparison of 18F-FDG PET with conventional imaging modalities in lymph node staging of head and neck cancer. *Eur J Nucl Med* 1998;25:1255–1260.

Benchaou M, Lehmann W, Slosman D, et al. The role of FDG-PET in preoperative assessment of N-staging in head and neck cancer. *Acta Otolartngol* 1996;116:332–335.

Brun E, Kjellen E, Tennvall J, et al. FDG PET studies during treatment: prediction of therapy outcome in head and neck squamous cell carcinoma. *Head Neck* 2002;24:127–135.

Chisin R, Macapinlac HA. The indications of FDG-PET in neck oncology. *Radiol Clin North Am* 2000;38:999–1012.

Goerres GW, Von Schulthess GK, Hany TF. Positron emission tomography and PET/CT of the head and neck: FDG uptake in normal anatomy, in benign lesions and in changes resulting from treatment. *AJR Am J Roentgenol* 2002;179:1337–43.

Greene FL, Page DL, Fleming ID, et al. *AJCC Cancer Staging Manual*, Sixth Edition. New York: Springer, 2002.

Greven KM, Keyes JW Jr, Williams DW III, McGuirt WF, Joyce WT III. Occult Primary tumors of the head and neck: lack of benefit from positron emission tomography imaging with 2-[F-18]fluoro-2-deoxy-D-glucose. *Cancer* 1999;86:114–118.

Halfpenny W, Hain SF, Biassoni L, Maisey MN, Sherman JA, McGurk M. FDG-PET: a possible prognostic factor in head and neck cancer. Br J Cancer 2002;86:512–516.

Hannah A, Scott AM, Tochon-Danguy H, et al. Evaulation of 18 F-fluorodeoxyglucose positron emission tomography and computed tomography with histopathologic correlation in the initial staging of head and neck cancer. *Ann Surg* 2002;236:208–217.

Hustinx R, Smith RJ, Benard F, et al. Dual time point fluorine-18 fluorodeoxyglucose positron emission tomography: a potential method to differentiate malignancy from inflammation and normal tissue in the head and neck. *Eur J Nucl Med* 1999;26:1345–1348.

Johansen J, Eigtved A, Buchwald C, et al. Implication of 18F-flouro-2-deoxy-D-glucose positron emission tomography on management of carcinoma of unknown primary in the head and neck: a Danish cohort study. *Laryngoscope* 2002; 112:2009–14.

Kole AC, Nieweg OE, Pruim J, et al. Detection of unknown occult primary tumors using positron emission tomography. *Cancer* 1998;82:1160–1166.

Kostakoglu L, Goldsmith SJ. PET in the assessment of therapy response in patients with carcinoma of the head and neck and of the esophagus. *J Nucl Med* 2004;45:56–68.

Kubota K, Yokoyama J, Yamaguchi K, et al. FDG-PET delayed imaging for the detection of head and neck cancer recurrence after chemoradiotherapy: comparison with MRI/CT. *Eur J Nucl Med Mol Imaging* 2004;4:590–595.

Lowe VJ, Dunphy FR, Varvares M, et al. Evaluation of chemotherapy response in patients with advanced head and neck cancer using [F-18]fluorodeoxyglucose positron emission tomography. *Head Neck* 1997;19:666–674.

Peng N, Yen S, Liu W, Tsay D, Liu R. Evaluation of the effect of radiation therapy to nasopharyngeal carcinoma by positron emission tomography with fluorodeoxyglucose. *Clin Posit Imag* 2000;3:51–56.

Porceddu SV, et al. Utility of positron emission tomography for the detection of disease in residual neck nodes after (chemo)radiotherapy in head and neck cancer. *Head Neck* 2005;27(3):175–181.

Schoder H, Yeung HW. Positron emission imaging of head and neck cancer, including thyroid carcinoma. *Semin Nucl Med* 2004;34:180–197.

Schoder H, Yeung HW, Gonen M, Kraus D, Larson SM. Head and neck cancer: clinical usefulness and accuracy of PET/CT image fusion. *Radiology* 2004;231:65–7.

Schwartz DL, Rajendran J, Yueh B, et al. FDG-PET prediction of head and neck squamous cell cancer outcomes. Arch Otolaryngol Head Neck Surg 2004;130:1361–1367.

Stuckensen T, Kovacs AF, Adams S, Baum RP. Staging of the neck in patients with oral cavity squamous cell carcinomas: a prospective comparison of PET, ultrasound, CT and MRI. *J Craniomaxillofac Surg* 2000;28:319–324.

Terhaard CH, Bongers V, van Rijk PP, Hordijk GJ. F-18-fluoro-deoxyglucose positron-emission tomography scanning in detection of local recurrence after radiotherapy for laryngeal/pharyngeal cancer. *Head Neck* 2001;23:933–941.

Wong RJ, Lin DT, Schoder H, et al. Diagnostic and prognostic value of [(18)F]fluorodeoxyglucose positron emission tomography for recurrent head and neck squamous cell carcinoma. *J Clin Oncol* 2002;20:4199–4208.

Yen RF, Hung RL, Pan MH, et al. 18-fluoro-2-deoxyglucose positron emission tomography in detecting recurrent/residual nasopharyngeal carcinoma and comparison with MRI. *Cancer* 2003;98:283–287.

CHAPTER 7

Abella-Columna E, Valk PE. Positron emission tomography imaging in melanoma and lymphoma. *Semin Roentgenol* 2002;37:129–139.

Ackland KM, O'Doherty MJ, Russell-Jones R. The value of positron emission tomography scanning in the detection of subclinical metatatic melanoma. *J Am Acad Dermatol* 2000;42:606–611.

Argenyi EE, Dogan AS, Urdaneta LF et al. Detection of unsuspected metastases in a melanoma patient with positron emission tomography. *Clin Nucl Med* 1995;20:744.

Belhocine T, Pierard G, De Labrassine M, et al. Staging of regional nodes in AJCC stage I and II melanoma:18FDG PET imaging versus sentinal node detection. *Oncologist* 2002;7:271–278.

Eigtved A, Andersson AP, Dahlstrom K, et al. Use of fluorine-18 fluorodeoxyglucose positron emission tomography in the detection of silent metastases from malignant melanoma. *Eur J Nucl Med* 2000;27:70–75.

Finkelstein SE, Carrasquillo JA, Hoffman JM, et al. A prospective analysis of positron emission tomography and conventional imaging for detection of stage IV metastatic melanoma in patients undergoing metastasectomy. *Ann Surg Oncol* 2004;11:731.

Friedman KP, Wahl RL. Clinical use of positron emission tomography in the management of cutaneous melanoma. *Semin Nucl Med* 2004;34:242–253.

Fuster D, Chiang S, Johnson G, Schuchter LM, Zhuang H, Alavi A. Is 18F-FDG PET more accurate than standard diagnostic procedures in the detection of suspected recurrent melanoma? *J Nucl Med* 2004;45:1323–1327.

Greene FL, Page DL, Fleming ID, et al. *AJCC Cancer Staging Manual*, Sixth Edition. New York: Springer, 2002.

Holder WD Jr, White RL Jr, Zuger JH, Easton EJ Jr, Greene FL. Effectiveness of positron emission tomography for the detection of melanoma metastases. *Ann Surg* 1998;227:764–769.

Longo MI, Lazaro P, Bueno C, et al. Fluorodeoxyglucose positron emission tomography imaging versus sentinal node biopsy an the primary staging of melanoma patients. *Dermatol Surg* 2003;29:245–248.

Mijnhout GS, Hoekstra OS, van Tulder MW, Teule GJ, Deville WL. Systematic review of the diagnostic accuracy of (18)F-fluorodeoxyglucose positron emission tomography in melanoma patients. *Cancer* 2001;91:1530–1542.

Paquet P, Henry F, Belhocine T, et al. An appraisal of 18-flourodeoxyglucose positron emission tomography for melanoma staging. *Dermatology* 2000;200:167–169.

Prichard RS, Hill AD, Skehan SJ, O'Higgins NJ. Positron emission tomography for staging and management of malignant melanoma. *Br J Surg* 2002;89:389–396.

Schroder H, Larson SM, Yeung HW. PET/CT in oncology: integration into clinical management of lymphoma, melanoma and gastrointestinal malignancies. *J Nucl Med* 2004;45 Suppl 1:72S–81S.

Stas M, Stroobants S, Dupont P, et al. 18-FDG PET scan in the staging of recurrent melanoma: additional value and therapeutic impact. *Melanoma Res* 2002;12:479–490.

Wagner JD, Schauwecker D, Davidson D, et al. FDG-PET sensitivity for melanoma lymph node metastases is dependent on tumor volume. *J Surg Oncol* 2001;77:237–242.

Wagner JD, Schauwecker D, Davidson D, et al. Prospective study of fluorodeoxyglucose-positron emission tomography imaging of lymph node basins in melanoma patients undergoing sentinal node biopsy. *J Clin Oncol* 1999;17:1508–1515.

CHAPTER 8

Belhocine T, Thille A, Fridman V, et al. Contribution of whole-body 18FDG PET imaging in the management of cervical cancer. *Gynecol Oncol* 2002;87:90–97.

Belhocine TZ. 18F-FDG PET imaging in posttherapy monitoring of cervical cancers: from diagnosis to prognosis. *J Nucl Med* 2004;45:1602–1604.

Berchuk A, Boente MP, Bast RC Jnr. The use of tumour markers in the management of patients with gynaecological carcinomas. *Clin Obstet Gynecol* 1992;35:45–54.

Fenchel S, Grab D, Nuessle K, et al. Asymptomatic adnexal masses: correlation of FDG PET and histopathologic findings. *Radiology* 2002;223: 780–788.

Greene FL, Page DL, Fleming ID, et al. *AJCC Cancer Staging Manual*, Sixth Edition. New York: Springer, 2002.

Grigsby PW, Siegel BA, Dehdashti F. Lymph node staging by positron emission tomography in patients with carcinoma of the cervix. *J Clin Oncol* 2001;19:3745–3749.

Grigsby PW, Siegel BA, Dehdashti F, Mutch DG. Posttherapy surveillance monitoring of cervical cancer by FDG-PET. *Int J Radiat Oncol Biol Phys* 2003;55:907–913.

Hain SF, O'Doherty MJ, Timothy AR, et al. Fluorodeoxyglucose-PET in the evaluation of germ cell tumours at relapse. *Br J Cancer* 2000;83: 863–869.

Hain SF, O'Doherty MJ, Timothy AR et al. Fluorodeoxyglucose-PET in the initial staging of germ cell tumours. *Eur J Nucl Med* 2000;27: 590–594.

Havrilesky LJ, Kulasingam SL, Matchar DB, Myere ER. FDG-PET for management of cervical and ovarian cancer. *Gynecol Oncol* 2005 (1):183–191.

Hubner KF, McDonald TW, Niethammer JG, Smith GT, Gould HR, Buonocore E. Assessment of primary and metastatic ovarian cancer by positron emission tomography (PET) using 2-[18F]deoxyglucose (2-[18F]FDG). *Gynecol Oncol* 1993;51:197–204.

Lai CH, Huang KG, See LC et al. Restaging of recurrent cervical carcinoma with dual-phase [18F]fluoro-2-deoxy-D-glucose positron emission tomography. *Cancer* Feb 1, 2004;100(3):544–552.

Lassen U, Daugaard G, Eigtved A et al. Whole body FDG-PET in patients with stage I non-seminomatous germ cell tumours. *Eur J Nucl Med Mol Imaging* 2005;30:396–402.

Lerman H, Metser U, Grisaru D, Fishman A, Lievshitz G, Even-Sapir E. Normal and abnormal 18F-FDG endometrial and ovarian uptake in pre- and post-menopausal patients: assessment by PET/CT. *J Nucl Med* 2004;45:266–271.

Lin WC, Hung YC, Yeh LS, Kao CH, Yen RF, Shen YY. Usefulness of (18)F-fluorodeoxyglucose positron emission tomography to detect para-aortic lymph nodal metastasis in advanced cervical cancer with negative computed tomography findings. *Gynecol Oncol* 2003;89: 73–76.

Ma SY, See LC, Lai CH, et al. Delayed (18)F-FDG PET for detection of paraaortic lymph node metastases in cervical cancer patients. *J Nucl Med* 2003;44:1775–1783.

Miller TR, Pinkus E, Dehdashti F, Grigsby PW. Improved prognostic value of 18F-FDG PET using a simple visual analysis of tumor characteristics in patients with cervical cancer. *J Nucl Med* 2003;44:192–197.

Narayan K, Hicks RJ, Jobling T, Bernshaw D, McKenzie AF. A comparison of MRI and PET scanning in surgically staged loco-regionally advanced cervical cancer: potential impact on treatment. *Int J Gynecol Cancer* 2001;11:263–271.

Reinhardt MJ, Ehritt-Braun C, Vogelgesang D, et. al. Metastatic lymph nodes in patients with cervical cancer: detection with MR imaging and FDG PET. *Radiology* 2001;218:776–782.

Reinhardt MJ, Ehritt-Braun C, Vogelgesang D, et al. Metastatic lymph nodes in patients with cervical cancer: detection with MR imaging and FDG PET. *Radiology* 2001;218(3):776–782.

Reinhardt MJ, Ehritt-Braun C, Vogelgesang D, et al. Metastatic lymph nodes in patients with cervical cancer: detection with MR imaging and FDG PET. *Radiology* 2001;218(3):776–782.

Rose PG, Adler LP, Rodriguez M, Faulhaber PF, Abdul-Karim FW, Miraldi F. Positron emission tomography for evaluating para-aortic nodal metastasis in locally advanced cervical cancer before surgical staging: a surgicopathologic study. *J Clin Oncol* 1999;17:41–45.

Ryu SY, Kim MH, Choi SC, Choi CW, Lee KH. Detection of early recurrence with 18F- FDG PET in patients with cervical cancer. *J Nucl Med* 2003;44:347–352.

Tempany CM, Zou KH, Silverman SG, et al. Staging of advanced ovarian cancer: comparison of imaging modalities—report from the Radiological Diagnostic Oncology Group. *Radiology* 2000;215:761–767.

Tsai CS, Chang TC, Lai CH, et al. Preliminary report of using FDG-PET to detect extrapelvic lesions in cervical cancer patients with enlarged pelvic lymph nodes on MRI/CT. *Int J Radiat Oncol Biol Phys* 2004;58:1506–1512.

Unger JB, Ivy JJ, Connor P, et al. Detection of recurrent cervical cancer by whole-body FDG PET scan in asymptomatic and symptomatic women. *Gynecol Oncol* 2004;94(1):212–216.

Unger JB, Ivy JJ, Connor P, et al. Detection of recurrent cervical cancer by whole-body FDG PET scan in asymptomatic and symptomatic women. *Gynecol Oncol* 2004;94(1):212–216.

Yen TC, See LC, Chang TC, et al. Defining the priority of using 18F-FDG PET for recurrent cervical cancer. *J Nucl Med* 2004;45:1632–1639.

Yoshida Y, Kurokawa T, Kawahara K, et al. Metabolic monitoring of advanced uterine cervical cancer neoadjuvant chemotherapy by using [F-18]-fluorodeoxyglucose positron emission tomography: preliminary results in three patients. *Gynecol Oncol* 2004;95:597–602.

CHAPTER 9

Asad S, Aquino SL, Piyavisetpat N, Fischman AJ. False-positive FDG positron emission tomography uptake in nonmalignant chest abnormalities. *AJR Am J Roentgenol* 2004;182:983–989.

Barrington SF, Maisey MN. Skeletal muscle uptake of fluorine-18-FDG: effect of oral diazepam. *J Nucl Med* 1996;37(7):1127–1129.

Chen YK, Chen YL, Liao AC, Shen YY, Kao CH. Elevated 18F-FDG uptake in skeletal muscles and thymus: a clue for the diagnosis of Grave's disease. *Nucl Med Commun* 2004;25:115–121.

Cohade C, Mourtzikos KA, Wahl RL. "USA-Fat": prevalence is related to ambient outdoor temperature-evaluation with 18F-FDG PET/CT. *J Nucl Med* 2003;44:1267–1270.

Cohade C, Osman M, Pannu HK, et al. Uptake in supraclavicular area fat: description on 18F-FDG PET/CT. *J Nucl Med* 2003;44:170–176.

Cook GJ, Fogelman I, Maisey MN. Normal physiological and benign pathological variants of 18-Flouro-2-Deoxyglucose positron-emission tomography scanning: potential for error in interpretation. *Semin Nucl Med* 1996;26(4):308–314.

Cook GJ, Maisey MN, Fogelman I, Normal variants, artefacts and interpretative pitfalls in PET imaging with 18-Flouro-2-Deoxyglucose and carbon-11 methionine. *Eur J Nucl Med* 1999;26(10):1363–1378.

Fayad LM, Cohade C, Wahl RL, Fishman EK. Sacral fractures: a potential pitfall of FDG positron emission tomography. *AJR Am J Roentgenol* 2003;181:1239–1243.

Ferdinand B, Gupta P, Kramer EL. Spectrum of thymic uptake at 18F-FDG PET. *Radiographics* 2004;24:1611–1616.

Gordon BA, Flanagan FL, Dehdashti F. Whole body positron emission tomography: normal variations, pitfalls and technical considerations. *AJR Am J Roentgenol* 1997;169(6):1675–1680.

Goerres GW, Ziegler SI, Burger C, Berthold T, Von Schulthess GK, Buck A. Artifacts at PET and PET/CT caused by metallic hip prosthetic material. *Radiology* 2003:226:577–584.

Heller MT, Meltzer CC, Fukui MB et al. Supraphysiological FDG uptake in the non-paralyzed vocal cord. Resolution of a false positive PET result with combined PET-CT imaging. *Clin Positron Imaging* 2000; 3(5):207–211.

Kamel EM, Thumshirn M, Truninger K, et al. Significance of incidental 18F-FDG accumulations in the gastrointestinal tract in PET/CT: correlation with endoscopic and histopathologic results. *J Nucl Med* 2004; 45:1804–1810.

Koga H, Sasaki M, Kuwabara Y, et al. An analysis of the physiological FDG uptake pattern in the stomach. *Ann Nucl Med* 2003;17:733–738.

Nakahara T, Fujii H, Ide M, et al. FDG uptake in the physiologically normal thymus: comparison of FDG positron emission tomography and CT. *Br J Radiol* 2001;74(885):821–824.

Pandit-Taskar N, Sinha A, Gonen M, et al. Testicular uptake in 18FDG PET scan. *J Nucl Med* 2001;5(S):287P.

Shon IH, Fogelman I. F-18 FDG positron emission tomography and benign fractures. *Clin Nucl Med* 2003;28:171–175.

Shreve PD, Anzai Y, Wahl RL. Pitfalls in oncological diagnosis with FDG PET imaging: physiological and benign variants. *Radiographics* 1999; 19(1):61–77.

Shreve PD, Wahl RL. Normal variants in FDG PET imaging. In: RL Wahl, ed. Principles and practice of positron emission tomography. Philadelphia, PA: Lippincott Williams & Wilkins;2002:111–136.

Tatidil R, Jadvar H, Bading JR, Conti PS. Incidental colonic fluorodeoxyglucose uptake: correlation with colonoscopic and histopathologic findings. *Radiology* 2002;224(3):783–787.

Truong MT, Erasmus JJ, Munden RF, et al. Focal FDG uptake in mediastinal brown fat mimicking malignancy: a potential pitfall resolved on PET/CT. *AJR Am J Roentgenol* 2004;183:1127–1132.

Yeung HW, Grewal RK, Gonen M, Schoder H, Larson SM. Patterns of (18)F-FDG uptake in adipose tissue and muscle: a potential source of false-positives for PET. *J Nucl Med* 2003;44:1789–1796.

CHAPTER 10

Agress H Jr, Cooper BZ. Detection of clinically unexpected malignant and premalignant tumors with whole-body FDG PET: histopathologic comparison. *Radiology* 2004;230:417–422.

Bai C, Kinahan PE, Brasse D, et al. An analytic study of the effects of attenuation on tumor detection in whole-body PET oncology imaging. *J Nucl Med* 2003;44:1855–1861.

Beyer T, Townsend DW, Brun T, et al. A combined PET/CT scanner for clinical oncology. *J Nucl Med* 2000;41:1369–1379.

Bleckmann C, Dose J, Bohuslavizki KH, et al. Effect of attenuation correction on lesion detectability in FDG PET of breast cancer. *J Nucl Med* 1999;40:2021–2024.

Boellaard R, Krak NC, Hoekstra OS, Lammertsma AA. Effects of noise, image resolution, and ROI definition on the accuracy of standard uptake values: a simulation study. *J Nucl Med* 2004;45:1519–1527.

Bohnen N. Neurological applications. In: RL Wahl, ed. Principles and practice of positron emission tomography. Philadelphia, PA: Lippincott Williams & Wilkins;2002:276–297.

Cherry SR, Sorenson JA, Phelps ME. *Physics in Nuclear Medicine*, 3rd ed. Philadelphia: Saunders, 2003.

Conrad GR, Sinha P. Narrow time-window dual-point 18F-FDG PET for the diagnosis of thoracic malignancy. *Nucl Med Commun* 2003;24:1129–1137.

Dobert N, Hamscho N, Menzel C, Neuss L, Kovacs AF, Grunwald F. Limitations of dual time point FDG-PET imaging in the evaluation of focal abdominal lesions. *Nuklearmedizin* 2004;43:143–149.

Erdi YE, Nehmeh SA, Pan T, et al. The CT motion quantitation of lung lesions and its impact on PET-measured SUVs. *J Nucl Med* 2004;45:1287–1292.

Hoffman EJ, Phelps ME. *Positron emission tomography: principles and quantitation.* New York: Raven Press;1986: pp 237–286.

Jadvar H, Parker JA. *Clinical PET and PET/CT*: Springer 2005.

Jaskowiak CJ, Bianco JA, Perlman SB, Fine JP. Influence of reconstruction iterations on 18F-FDG PET/CT standardized uptake values. *J Nucl Med* 2005;46:424–428.

Nakamoto Y, Osman M, Cohade C, et al. PET/CT: comparison of quantitative tracer uptake between germanium and CT transmission attenuation-corrected images. *J Nucl Med* 2002;43:1137–1143.

Pandit-Taskar N, Schoder H, Gonen M, Larson SM, Yeung HW. Clinical significance of unexplained abnormal focal FDG uptake in the abdomen during whole-body PET. *AJR Am J Roentgenol* 2004;183: 1143–1147.

Schoder H, Erdi YE, Chao K, Gonen M, Larson SM, Yeung HW. Clinical implications of different image reconstruction parameters for interpretation of whole-body PET studies in cancer patients. *J Nucl Med* 2004;45:559–566.

Wahl RL. To AC or not to AC: that is the question. *J Nucl Med* 1999;40: 2025–2028.

Zasadny KR, Wahl RL. Standardized uptake values of normal tissues with FDG: variation with body weight and method for correction. *Radiology* 1993;189(3):847–850.

Index

Printed in Singapore